FLASHBACKS NO. 12

The Flashback series is sponsored by the
European Ethnological Research Centre,
c/o the Royal Museums of Scotland,
Chambers Street, Edinburgh EH1 1JF.

General Editor: Alexander Fenton

For David, with love

SCOTTISH MIDWIVES

Twentieth-Century Voices

Lindsay Reid

TUCKWELL PRESS
in association with
The European Ethnological Research Centre

First published in Great Britain in 2000 by
Tuckwell Press
The Mill House
Phantassie
East Linton
East Lothian EH40 3DG
Scotland

British Library Cataloguing in Publication Data
A catalogue record for this book is available
on request from the British Library

Typeset by Hewer Text Ltd, Edinburgh
Printed and bound by The Cromwell Press, Trowbridge, Wiltshire

CONTENTS

Acknowledgements   vii
Foreword by Professor Edith Hillan   ix
Explanation of Terms   xi

Introduction   1
1. Ann Lamb   11
2. Mima Sutherland   17
3. Margaret Foggie   22
4. Chrissie Sandison   29
5. Molly Muir   35
6. Annie Kerr   41
7. Doddie Davidson   45
8. From the Outer Hebrides   53
9. Anne Chapman   63
10. Alice May Brodie Porter   69
11. Ella Banks and Linda Stamp   72
12. Peggy Grieve   82
13. Anne Bayne   93
14. Ella Clelland   115
15. 'I'm Glad I Came Back'   126
16. Stuart Hislop   137
17. Elizabeth Carson   146
18. Alison Dale and Maureen Hamilton   157
19. Joan Spence   170
20. Raigmore Midwives: Ayleen Marshall,
    Nikki Morton, Greta Renwick, Joan Kelly   181

Acknowledgements

Firstly, I should like to thank all the people who have so readily given of their time and memories. Without them this book would not have been written and I greatly appreciate all the help they have given me. They are: Ann Lamb, Mima Sutherland, Margaret Foggie, Chrissie Sandison, Molly Muir (now deceased), Annie Kerr, Doddie Davidson, Anne Chapman, Alice Porter, Ella Banks, Linda Stamp, Peggy Grieve, Anne Bayne, Ella Clelland, Stuart Hislop, Elizabeth Carson, Alison Dale, Maureen Hamilton, Joan Spence, Ayleen Marshall, Nikki Morton, Greta Renwick, Joan Kelly and two midwives who have requested that their names should not be made public.

Finding midwives to interview was achieved through writing to the press and by word of mouth. I am indebted to all the Scottish publications who published my letters asking for contacts, and all who 'networked' for me. Beatrice Grant of the National Board for Scotland for Nurses, Midwives and Health Visitors and Anne Matthew, Glasgow Caledonian University, must have run up a large telephone bill on my behalf, and Helen Bryars, Head of Midwifery in Inverness went to great lengths to organise my Raigmore visit. I am very grateful.

Thank you also to Professor Edith Hillan, Professor of Midwifery at the University of Glasgow for agreeing so readily to write the Foreword to 'Scottish Midwives' and for her unfailing support and help.

I should also like to record my appreciation to Dr Marguerite Dupree and Dr Malcolm Nicholson, both of the Wellcome Unit for the History of Medicine, the University of Glasgow, for their interest and encouragement, not forgetting my fellow students at the Wellcome Unit especially Anne Cameron and Jenny Cronin.

Friends at the Royal College of Midwives Scottish Board, Edinburgh: Patricia Purton, Director, Margaret McGuire, Education and Research Officer, Helen Henderson, Business Manager and Evangeline Creighton who was Education Officer before she retired. I greatly appreciate their ever-present support. Thank you also to all my other midwife friends who have shown so much interest and especially to Claire Shearer for her constant encouragement and friendship.

Choosing a title proved to be problematic. Suggestions ranged from things midwives are known to say frequently, like, 'I can see the head', (son Ewan), 'Your baby's got ginger hair', (midwife Marianne McInally), 'Mrs Brown's fully dilated', (Mags McGuire), and other witticisms, to a phrase including a collective noun for midwives (is there one?) and titles like 'Midwives, mothers and babies'. Thank you to all who made suggestions.

Mrs Agnes Young very kindly sent me a copy of the photograph of her grandmother Mary Bryce Smellie Henderson a long time ago. I appreciated this at the time and even more so now that Agnes has so freely agreed to allow the photo to be used on the cover of 'Scottish Midwives'. Mary Henderson was one of the first midwives to be included in the Roll of Midwives kept from 1916 by the Central Midwives' Board for Scotland.

Thanks also to Dr John Tuckwell of Tuckwell Publishing Ltd. for helpful suggestions, guidance during the writing process and for taking *Scottish Midwives* on.

Lastly, I should like to thank my family, David, Ruth, Ewan and Robert for putting up with their daft mother during this gestation period and especially my husband David, for his long-suffering patience, ever-listening ear and ready advice.

FOREWORD

The history of childbirth over the last century is often portrayed as the gradual encroachment of medical men into what was once a female preserve. Certainly until the end of the nineteenth century in Scotland, childbirth largely took place in the home with the woman attended by a midwife or howdie. There was no legislation to govern midwifery practice and although some midwives were professionally trained, many had learned their craft through experience and practice.

The twentieth century saw many changes in the delivery of maternity care. The Midwives Act was passed in England in 1902 and was followed by the Midwives (Scotland) Act of 1915. These Acts put an end to the practice of uncertified midwives by making training, examination and registration for midwives compulsory. Although the purpose of the legislation was to make midwives safer birth attendants, some would argue that it brought about the decline of the midwifery by introducing increasing medical control of their practice.

Whatever the truth of these arguments, there is very little documentary evidence of how midwives felt about these changes and the impact they had on their practice. How midwives felt about their training and rules which now governed their practice is very much uncharted territory. They were also having to cope with other changes in the delivery of maternity care such as the shift away from home births towards hospital delivery, the rise of the obstetric profession and the medicalisation of childbirth.

Lindsay's book gives us a rich insight into the way that Scottish midwives felt and feel about their work and the changes which impacted on their working lives. By telling their tales, the midwives who contributed to the book have allowed us to share their experiences and emotions of what it was like to be a midwife thoughout the twentieth century. We have much to learn from their voices.

Edith Hillan
Professor of Midwifery
University of Glasgow

EXPLANATION OF TERMS

Amniocentesis a procedure where some of the fluid surrounding the fetus in utero is drawn off.

Anti-D a substance given to mothers who are Rhesus negative, after delivery or some procedures to prevent their absorbing any fetal red blood cells in their circulation.

ARM Artificial rupture of membranes.

At da faain fit getting near the time of delivery. (Shetland)

Bandl's ring constricting ring around the uterus which can develop in labour and which prevents labour from progressing.

Blue Book pupil midwife's case book required by the CMB for Part 2 midwifery.

Boyle's machine anaesthetic machine.

Breakfast test meal a test to determine the level of glucose in the blood.

Buccal pitocin a development in induction of labour where the mother sucked the ocytocic drug.

Caul the term used to describe the membranes when they are delivered with the baby and cover the face and head. It is considered by some to be extremely lucky, the belief being that if a baby is born with a caul on its face, it will never drown. Sometimes it was kept amongst family heirlooms as a charm.

CMB Central Midwives' Board, in this instance, for Scotland. The CMB was the statutory body for midwives from 1916-1983.

Co-op card a card carried by the mother, containing her details and the history of the current pregnancy, and which is completed at every antenatal examination by midwife or doctor.

CTG cardiotocograph. A way of measuring continuously the fetal heart rate and movements, and uterine activity.

CVS chorionic villus sample.

D&C dilatation and curettage.

DNS Director of Nursing Services.

DOMINO Domiciliary in and out – community midwife care for a hospital delivery and home six hours later.

Double-duty a person who works as a midwife and a nurse on the community. (See treble-duty)

Dunny dungeon, area under a tenement.

DVT deep vein thrombosis.

Eclampsia, pre-eclampsia serious conditions specific to pregnancy and childbirth.

Elective section Caesarean section done on a day planned in advance for an obstetric or medical reason.

Elsie's Elsie Inglis Memorial Hospital, Edinburgh.

Entonox inhalational analgesia comprising nitrous oxide and oxygen in a fifty-fifty mix.

Flat baby a baby who is born in poor condition.

Grading a system currently in use, determining the level of salary and status of midwives and nurses in the UK. The minimum grade for a registered nurse is D. The Royal College of Midwives currently recommends that, owing to the level of responsibility which a midwife undertakes, midwives should be graded at a minimum of F. This recommendation is not always followed.

Grande multiparous mother a mother who has had six or more pregnancies.

Green Lady Glasgow Municipal midwife.

Gyn gynaecology.

Higginson's syringe an old-fashioned syringe used for giving enemata and vaginal douches.

Hippit passed over, exempted, excused.

Integrated midwifery a system of maternity care where community midwives are closely linked with a maternity unit.

Maek, maik a ha-penny.

Matty Aberdeen Royal Maternity Hospital.

Explanation of Terms

Midwives' Bank a list of midwives who can be called upon if a maternity unit is short-staffed because of, e.g. staff illness, extra work-load.

MOF Ministry of Food.

Mouser moustache.

NCT National Childbirth Trust.

Oil, bath and enema, OBE an old method of inducing labour.

OP occipito posterior.

Os opening of the cervix.

Para in this context, describing the number of babies a woman has had e.g. para 1 = had 1 baby.

Parous describing a woman who has had a baby previously.

Peerie small.

PIH pregnancy induced hypertension.

PPH post partum haemorrhage.

Prem premature.

Prim, primigravida a mother who is pregnant for the first time.

Pseudocyesis false pregnancy.

Queen's, Queen's Nursing Training District nurse training run by the Queen's Institute for District Nurses.

Rooming in system of care in a maternity unit where babies stay with the mothers all the time.

Rotten Row Glasgow Royal Maternity Hospital.

Salmon (Report) name given to the Report of a Committee on Senior Nursing Staff Structure (1966) under the chairmanship of Mr Brian Salmon, and the subsequent restructuring of senior nursing and midwifery staff in the UK.

SCBU Special Care Baby Unit.

Shared care antenatal care which is shared between community and hospital staff.

SHO Senior House Officer.

Skye accident a fatal accident which happened in December 1993 in icy conditions on the road between Skye and Inverness while a mother in labour was being transported to the Maternity Unit at Raigmore Hospital, Inverness. The midwife and paramedic were killed and some time later, the woman gave birth to a stillborn baby.

Simpson's Simpson Memorial Maternity Pavilion, Edinburgh.

Slippery elm the mucilaginous bark of the tree 'slippery elm' was used medicinally to soothe and help irritation.

Slunge, slungeing terms used in hospitals to describe work done in the sluice area of a ward.

Straw-box old-fashioned incubator.

Syntocinon artificial oxytocin used intravenously to induce or augment labour.

Syntometrine a drug comprising syntocinon and ergometrine used to assist and speed up the third stage of labour.

Term forty weeks pregnant. Often used to cover the period from thirty-seven or thirty-eight weeks to forty-two weeks.

Treble duty a person who works as midwife, nurse and health visitor on the community.

VE vaginal examination.

Ventouse a method of delivering a baby where the mother is assisted by the use of a vacuum extractor placed on the fetal head.

Vernix a creamy protective substance covering a fetus' body *in utero*.

Wheen quite a number.

Winchester large bottle often used for holding medicines, disinfectants etc. in bulk.

INTRODUCTION

There is little written about midwives in Scotland in the twentieth century. I discovered this when I was trying to find out some of the background to the changes that were happening to midwifery practice and education in the 1990s. The search was so frustrating that I decided to do something about it.

I wrote to many Scottish newspapers and other publications asking for help. The response was just what I wanted. Letters and phone calls came from midwives all over Scotland volunteering to tell their story and encouraging me to get on with it. Not only that, the word spread as one told another. Now I have an increasingly thick file of names, contacts and stories and I am sure there are more to come.

Of course, midwives do not belong only to the twentieth century. There have always been midwives in Scotland. However, many twentieth-century midwives are still here to tell their stories for themselves and this is how this book has come about. To set the scene and put their stories in context, I am including here a short section on what went before.

The term 'midwife' is very old and is commonly understood to mean 'the with-woman' – that is, the woman who is with a mother in childbirth. However, they were not always called midwives – the favourite old name is *howdie*. This is universally understood across Scotland but has variations depending on the area. *Howdie wife* was commonly heard and in the North East you might find a further diminutive giving *howdie wifie*. Elsewhere you would hear other terms being used like *skilly* or *skilful woman, handy woman, neighbour woman, helping woman.* On the Island of St. Kilda the term *bean-glhuine* or *knee woman* was used, and elsewhere in the Highlands the Gaelic *ban chuideachaidh,* literally meaning 'aid woman', would be used

Many midwives came to their profession by chance. Attendance at one birth with an existing midwife would lead to being asked to attend another birth. Skill was built up by practical experience and a midwife in an area became established by reputation. She was usually a respected figure, usually had borne children herself, was perhaps a widow, but had no formal training and no particular knowledge of cleanliness and hygiene.

Chrissie Sandison, from Aith, in Shetland, remembers hearing about howdies:

> I had a grand-aunt who was the age I am now [80] when I was a teenager. She had had no children of her own, never was married, a peerie body who was in attendance at many a birth. I asked her how it was she had taken up to be a howdie for she had had no proper training. Apparently, her mother Hannah had been a howdie and when she began to get old she began taking Meggie along too, so . . . There were big families in those days – that would have been from about 1880 onwards. This Meggie had been born in 1858 and was in attendance at the birth of one of my nephews in 1926.

Until the twentieth century there was no legislation in Britain governing midwifery practice. Before the mid-eighteenth century, midwives, mostly untrained, were the people expected to care for and deliver women in childbirth and call for a male medical practitioner in an emergency. From the mid-eighteenth century, the presence of male practitioners in the delivery room became more common even for normal births. Men dominated the training of midwives as well, and as time went on more midwives undertook a form of training supervised by medical practitioners. The first training school for midwives in the United Kingdom was established in Edinburgh in 1726 when the Town Council appointed Joseph

Introduction

Gibson Professor of Midwifery. A similar midwifery training school was established in Glasgow in December 1739 under the auspices of the Faculty of Physicians and Surgeons in Glasgow. Other midwifery training schools followed in both Scotland and England. However, throughout Britain there was no uniformity of midwifery training and nothing to regularise it. In addition, any woman was able to practise midwifery, and the untrained midwife was more commonly seen than otherwise, especially amongst less well-off child-bearing women.

Registration of midwives was opposed for many years by members of the General Medical Council, particularly general practitioners (GPs).[1] The main reason for this was that the medical profession saw competition from midwives becoming greater if midwives were to be registered and their training regulated. However, the opposing argument was that, with more education, more midwives would recognise the abnormal and more midwives would therefore call medical aid. Also, GPs saw midwifery as a way of expanding their practice. If they attended the mother in childbirth, the odds were that they could claim the rest of the family as patients too.

Finally, after twenty years of effort[2] the first Midwives Act was passed in 1902 and arrangements were made for the registration of midwives in England and Wales but not for Scotland and Ireland. This was a major landmark in the professionalisation of midwifery and for the mothers and infants they cared for.

The Midwives (Scotland) Act followed in 1915. Dr. A.K. Chalmers, the then Medical Officer of Health for Glasgow, felt strongly that for the sake of mothers and babies in Scotland maternity care should be improved and supervised.[3] He was a key figure in the campaign to have a Scottish Midwives Bill.

After much campaigning and agitating, towards the end of 1915, during the First World War, legislation for midwives in Scotland looked as though it was going to become a reality. At the second reading of the Bill in the Commons on 25

3

Scottish Midwives

November 1915, introduced by Mr McKinnon Wood MP, the urgency of the need for a Midwives Bill for Scotland was made clear. 'A great many representations have been made to me by practically [all] the heads of the medical profession, and also by public health authorities and others, that in this time of war there was a special need for a Bill of this kind.'[4] Mr McKinnon Wood said that he had been approached by representatives from the medical profession, public health authorities and the Principal of Glasgow University making a case for a Midwives Act for Scotland:

> As the House is aware, the medical profession has been sadly depleted. A great many doctors have gone to the front, leaving rural districts inadequately provided with medical practitioners; so that competent midwives are absolutely necessary throughout Scotland . . . The Scottish midwife is not able to obtain a formal qualification except in England Altogether, I think, the case for treating this as a matter of urgency is virtually made out on very high authority indeed.[5]

The Midwives (Scotland) Bill received Royal Assent on 23 December 1915[6] and the Act was implemented in January 1916. It made provision for the constitution of the Central Midwives' Board for Scotland (CMB). It was the Board's responsibility to implement measures to fulfil the aim of the Act 'to secure the better training of Midwives in Scotland, and to regulate their practice'.[7] The 1915 Act and similar subsequent Acts provided the statutory framework pertaining to midwives and maternity care in Scotland until 1983 when the Nurses, Midwives, and Health Visitors Act 1979 was implemented.

The Board had the power to frame rules under the 1915 Midwives (Scotland) Act and to see that these were upheld. The Rules covered all aspects of midwifery in Scotland and were updated regularly. They covered the proceedings of the Board, regulated the issue of certificates to midwives and the care of the Roll of Midwives. They regulated the training of midwives and the conduct of examinations. At the very beginning of the CMB's work they had to decide on the admission to the Roll

4

of women who were already practising. These midwives could be certificated already by means of a hospital training at one of a list of specifically approved hospitals. Also, midwives who had been in 'bona fide' practice for a minimum of a year, but who did not hold a certificate from a recognised hospital or body, could also be registered provided they were 'trustworthy, sober and of good moral character'.[8]

One of the main objectives of the Midwives (Scotland) Act 1915 was to put an end to the practice of uncertified midwives. After a year's grace no woman could call herself a midwife without being certified under the Act. Also, after 1 January 1922, no woman in Scotland 'shall habitually and for gain attend women in childbirth otherwise than under the direction of a registered medical practitioner unless she be certified under this Act'.[9] The use of the term, 'habitually and for gain', which appeared in both the English and the Scottish Acts, was controversial[10] as it allowed uncertified women to practise as midwives as long as it could be seen that they were not doing it 'habitually and for gain'. This left a loophole in the law which official bodies were anxious to close.

The law about unqualified midwives was made progressively stricter with first the 1927 Midwives and Maternity Homes (Scotland) Act which got rid of the 'habitually and for gain' phrase and then the 1937 Maternity Services (Scotland) Act which addressed the question of women who were neither certified midwives nor registered nurses and who were paid to look after women in childbirth and in the fourteen days afterwards.

However, many medical practitioners and uncertified midwives or howdies worked together successfully. As far as the mothers were concerned, the howdies were popular as they were cheaper than the certified midwives, and would stay in the home with the family from before the birth until at least two weeks afterwards and do far more in the way of housework like cleaning, baking and cooking than a midwife would. Not only that, the medical practitioners appeared to like working with them – indeed uncertified midwives who worked in this way depended on the GPs as well as word of mouth for work.

Howdies, neighbour-women, skilly women, unqualified midwives – call them what you like – were a very important part of life in Scottish families in the first half of the twentieth century. They are remembered with affection and for the caring they brought to the work they did. Two of them are described in the following letters.

Johnann Roberton

I am 62 years old. Born 27.09.34.

I was born in Aberdeen City at home.

I was delivered by my grandmother – Johnann Roberton who was the uncertificated midwife for the King Street and surrounding streets. She was employed by a Dr. Coutts who I believe was specialising in confinements and child care.

He ran the main surgery in King Street and she was called out at all hours to confinements in houses.

She had her own special "BAG" and on her pre-natal visits she instructed the mothers on what she would need regarding equipment at the time of birth and I believe that she was a stickler for having everything ready in advance wherever possible in those days.

When a birth happened unexpectedly, Dr. Coutts would collect her in his little car but otherwise she had to walk to all the other call-outs. She liked to be summoned in the first stages of labour to avoid complications where possible and lived and worked by the idea that 'To be forewarned was to be forearmed'.

Postnatally

She had a strict routine and according to my late mother, Granma would clean up the patient first after the expulsion of the afterbirth and immediately wrap her up in a supporting binder round the stomach top prevent sagging of the abdominal muscles. My mother felt the benefit of this in later years!

The binders were usually made of flannelette sheets torn to the required strips for size. She also collected old sheets from neighbours and made the bandages herself. If the mother had insufficient milk, her breasts were "binded" too to prevent drooping.

Her fees varied from house to house and of course she rarely got paid by the Doctor and only in difficult or long cases did she get a shilling or two. But her patients sometimes paid her in kind, e.g. eggs, bread etc.

She had twelve children herself in all – three neo-natal deaths, three sons died young, two daughters died in their seventies, but my two remaining youngest late baby aunts are now in their eighties and going strong.

She was only 5ft. 2inches in height and although she'd had all those children she continued to work until about 1936. [One year before the Maternity Services (Scotland) Act.] She was born in 1871 and died 86 years later, outliving the doctor she'd worked for.

You will see, therefore, that although midwifery was legalised in 1916 the howdie wifie was still active in this area for another twenty years.

Letter from Moira Michie.

Margaret Anderson Watson

Although I now live in England, I was born in the parish of Douglas, Lanarkshire, in 1911.

My Grandfather was signalman at Douglas Station (later re-named Happendon) from 1877 to 1924. Between these dates until 1923 when she died, my Grandmother, Margaret Anderson Watson, was the Howdie for the Happendon area.

Happendon Station, now closed, was in the heart of Happendon Woods, where, in the old days, there were small encampments for tinkers with their horse caravans and makeshift tents.

They would stay a few days to sell their pots and pans and conveniently, on many occasions, long enough for the wives to avail themselves of my Grandmother's services.

I wrote the enclosed poem in February 1994, inspired by hearing some reference to Howdies in general:

GRAN – THE HOWDIE OF HAPPENDON!

When I was a boy and staying with Gran,
There came to the door a young tinker man,
In the early hours of a winter morn.
And said: 'My bairn will sune be born,
Could ye come wi me to Cock-ma-lane,
And help the wife tae hae the wean?'

In case the lass was in distress,
Gran took her black bag from the press
And off on that frosty morn she went,
To help the wife in the tinker's tent.
And there in the moonlight's fleeting beam,
The bairn was born and washed in the stream.

For Gran was the tinkers' Howdie wife,
To them she could mean a death or a life,
And many a tinker bairn came good,
She had brought to life in Happenden Wood.

Each one of the gangrel tinker clan,
Greatly respected our kindly Gran,
Not one her hens or eggs would steal,
They'd rather do without a meal.

They gave no payment for her task,
No payment did she ever ask.
But always at her cottage door,
They left her with pans for evermore!

When Springtime cleared their aches and pains,
And wanderlust got in their veins,
At Gran's they shed a farewell tear,
And said they'd meet, same time next year.

Letter from James W. Tweedie.

Introduction

As the number of certified midwives increased, the number of howdies diminished. The CMB developed from a new body, feeling its way, to an influential group which kept a close watch on midwifery and maternity care in Scotland until the 1979 Nurses, Midwives and Health Visitors Act was implemented in 1983. Then the responsibility was handed over to the United Kingdom Central Council for Nurses, Midwives and Health Visitors and four National Boards, one for each country of the United Kingdom.

Through the twentieth century midwives have coped with many changes – in practice and education, with poverty and depression, with War and the coming of the National Health Service. They have struggled for their existence, being dubbed many times 'the doctor's handmaiden', and have coped with over-medicalisation of maternity care. In the last decades of the century the tide has turned. Midwives, women and other professionals in the field have worked together for more informed choice for women, greater autonomy for midwives and more sensible use of the many technological advances which have been made.

An oral history testimony gives a picture of how an individual remembers an incident, a decade, a career, a lifetime. In this book of oral history testimonies, midwives in Scotland tell the history of midwifery in Scotland in the twentieth century from their own, very personal perspectives.

Notes

1 J. Donnison, *Midwives and Medical Men* (New Barnet: Historical Publications, 1988), p.138.
2 B. Cowell, and D.Wainwright, *Behind the Blue Door. The History of the Royal College of Midwives 1881-1981* (London: Bailliere Tindall, 1981), p.33.
3 A. MacGregor, *Public Health in Glasgow 1905-1946* (Edinburgh and London: E.and S. Livingstone Ltd, 1967), p 110.
4 *Hansard*, Commons, Vol. 26, Nov 22-Dec 17 1915, col. 480.
5 *Hansard*, Commons, Vol. 26, Nov 22-Dec 17 1915, col. 480-481.
6 *Hansard,* Commons, Vol. 27, Dec 23 1915, col. 806.

Scottish Midwives

7 *Midwives (Scotland) Act*, 1915 [5 & 6 Geo. 5. Ch. 91] Section 1, p 3.
8 NAS, CMB 4/2/10, *CMB Rules*, p. 7.
9 *Midwives (Scotland) Act*, 1915, Section 1 (2).
10 Hansard, Commons, Vol. 26, Nov 22-Dec 17, 1915, col.482.

I

ANN LAMB

Ann Lamb was born in Glenlivet in 1902. She trained as a midwife in Edinburgh before doing nurse training. She worked for many years as midwife and nurse in Scotland and delivered many babies.

In her later years Ann wrote a book of her life, some of which was hand-written and some recorded. Although the book has not been published in its entirety, an extract has been published in 'Tales of the Braes of Glenlivet' (Birlinn, 1999). Ann has given permission for further extracts about her career in midwifery to be used here to augment her oral testimony. She now lives in a Nursing Home in Stonehaven.

Ann's prizewinning poem, written when she was at the Royal Infirmary of Edinburgh, begins her story:

The World grows better year by year
Because some nurse in her little sphere
Puts on her apron and grins and sings
And keeps on doing the same old things.
Feeding the patients and answering the bells,
And doing the things that her heart rebels.
Blessing the newborn babe's first breath.
Closing the eyes that are still in death.
Taking the blame for the Doctors' mistakes
Oh dear what a lot of patience it takes.
Going off duty at eight o'clock
Discouraged and tearful and ready to drop.
Called back for a special at 8.15
With woe in her heart but must *not* be seen.
Morning and evening noon and night,
Just doing it over and hoping it's right.

I belong to Glenlivet. I was brought into the world on 25th February 1902, probably by Meg Gordon the howdie, the midwife for the district, who liked a dram. I am told there were six feet of snow and because the roads were blocked, the doctor never saw me for six weeks. Doctors nowadays don't know what they're talking about. Talking about sepsis – there was no sepsis. People were self-taught and they were wonderful.

When I was in my twenties I was thinking about what to do. I met a girl who suggested nursing but I didn't think I would get in. She said, 'You would get into Edinburgh Royal if you have one certificate – midwifery'. She said there was a place where I could train and you got to the Canongate and the Cowgate and all the poor quarters. She introduced me to this doctor and he said, 'Oh, you'll get by, you're from the country', and so I went in. This wasn't the big place – the Simpson – but just up the road from it. It was small but you got a good training as a midwife. This was in 1927 and the training was a year, from 1927 to 1928. It wasn't long enough but we managed.

We stayed in the building and there were only about ten of us. We went to lots of classes because you never learned if you didn't go, and out on the district as well. It was a hard training . . . Sometimes you would be going down the street to see a woman and a head would pop out at the window. 'Oh nurse come and help me.' You had never seen her before, you didn't know her name, and up the stairs you went and delivered the baby. She would know who *you* were.

There was no antenatal care and poverty was very bad. It was terrible, they had no clothes, no nothing. You had to boil the water when you arrived for the delivery, and you carried everything in a black bag. We had no taxis and walked everywhere in all weathers. From Lauriston Place to the foot of the Lawnmarket, it was quite a step. They were very poor. There was only one sheet to deliver the mother on, so a firm was very good and gave us paper, white wallpaper, and we made a sheet of that. We had nothing much to work on, but I never remember a case of sepsis or anything wrong with the mother or baby. They were very happy but they had nothing. I just can't tell you what we witnessed during that time. It was terrible. There was a doctor who came if you were in distress about the delivery, but somehow it seemed the babies all just came out and there was no trouble. I probably did about two hundred deliveries on the district in Edinburgh. We were at it daily. They were nice, cheery people and were always glad to see us. I did the year and then I passed. So I finally got my Certificate of the Midwifery Board (Central Midwives Board) which I have to this day.

Then I got at last to Edinburgh Royal which had about five hundred beds at that time. In those days this was *the* hospital in Scotland. Aberdeen was only a wee place at Woolmanhill. I had to meet the Matron who was an utter snob. She interviewed me and she weighed me, asked a lot of questions, oh very very particular about that, and she said, 'Well you'll be taken on trial in the PTS which was the Preliminary Training School, for six weeks'. It was hard work. The Sister Tutor was a terror but excellent. I passed PTS with good marks and got in. I started in 1932 and trained till 1936. So then I was both a nurse and a midwife. My mother was very proud of me doing this. I was very happy. I was in Edinburgh Royal for five years. The pelican was the badge – I was a pelican. I also had a CMB badge.

I went to Aberdeen and joined an Association of Trained Nurses based at the Armstrong Nursing Home which is now St. John's. In those days there were three nursing homes in Aberdeen – Kepplestone, the Northern and the Armstrong. Miss Ross from Torphins was the Matron of the Armstrong. She was very strict and only took on nurses capable of going to Balmoral. I didn't want to go on the indoor staff. I had had enough of indoors. So she said, 'Oh well, I'll have to vet you first. I'm very particular about my outdoor staff'. She was a tyrant. She went through everything, who you were, what you were and so on before she took me on.

It was a good job but not much money. I met a lot of nice people there and I nursed Lady Farquhar and the Admiral. He was funny – he was an Admiral of the Fleet. He liked a dram. They were so nice to me. When I was kind of tired she would say, 'Go and put your feet up and ask for a drink. Say I said so'.

I had hundreds of babies – sometimes more than you wanted. Sometimes there was a doctor there and sometimes not and I just had to do it. I was a good midwife. I managed fine.

One time I went to a house in Leven in Fife. The woman was very large. I was relieving the district nurse and she said, 'I think it's twins'. I said that it looked more like triplets. We had a laugh about it and she went away. The night I was called out to this woman in labour, the doctor was, of course, late as usual and the mother said, 'I hear I'm going to have twins'. I said, 'I hear three heart-beats. You've more than two, you've three'. She said, 'The Doctor won't be here'. Sure enough, I delivered two and then the third one. So, I delivered triplets, at home by myself. The births went very well. There was Errol and Pearl and John and they were all fine except that John was cramped a bit. He needed attention and we sent him to St. Andrews to the wee hospital there. No trouble at all. It was nothing in those days. You had to get on with it. She had five children before she had the triplets. I had two or three twin deliveries but not that many. Mostly single babies. I went from place to place to deliver them.

A month after the Fife triplets were born, I went to a job in Edinburgh. The head of the nursing home where I was on night duty said there was a lady going to have triplets. It was quite unusual to deliver two lots in one year. A doctor arrived who I immediately recognised as Professor Johnstone. He leaned over a chair and he said to me, 'Carry on'. I was terrified that anything would go wrong. He stayed, along with another midwife, and we delivered them. So I've had two sets of triplets. Nowadays if there is one set of triplets there's about eighteen doctors and seven or eight sisters and what a fuss. Fuss isn't normal, no trouble with babies at all.

I usually stayed in the house after the birth, sometimes a week but sometimes longer. That was for postnatal care but there wasn't really much postnatal care in my day – just a wee look. We saw to the baby too, bathing and feeding and looking after the cord. At birth, we stripped it, and tied it then cut it. We put a binder on it and took the binder off every day to wash it. We usually put a penny on the cord stump under the binder.

It was nice being at the birth. There was no antenatal care. Some people didn't even know they were having a baby till they delivered. But I was always quick on the draw. I carried my bag around with me – a brown bag. The mothers had to get things for the baby.

I had a second-hand bicycle which cost 2/6 (12½ pence). When they wanted me they phoned or came on a bicycle. Then I would go on my bicycle. I worked sometimes in Banchory. I stayed there waiting for the babies that arrived and I would go and deliver the baby. I delivered most of my babies at home without a doctor. Sometimes the doctors came and sometimes not. I felt safer with a doctor but I would still deliver the baby. The doctor was just there to look on. One of the Banchory doctors was Dr Emslie and I knew Dr. Park too. Once the mothers were in labour we never left them. It wouldn't do. I once had a book, a register, and kept the names but I don't know where it went to. Everybody knew me – Lambie.

I did district nursing in Ballater for a little time and liked that very much. I rode the bicycle. I was a great lass on the bicycle and I had fun. When the other war broke out I was still there. You had to agree to do midwifery as well as your other work or you got called up. So I was at the Castle, and Grantown-on-Spey at the hospital, down at Montrose, at Carnoustie, in Kirkcaldy. I don't think there is a town I haven't been in but not the west-coast towns – Oban and around there.

I was coming more or less nearer my retirement and I took a post as a midwifery sister in a small hospital in Banffshire with only five midwives. It was great, we had grand midwives. They were excellent and deliveries were nothing at all. I well remember women from the Cabrach coming in.

I also delivered all the going-about people, the Johnstones and all the people up north. They used to come to Huntly and live in the Market Square. They never had any antenatal and you never knew what was going to happen but everything was all right. They were the travelling people. I've had a lovely time.

2

MIMA SUTHERLAND

Mima Sutherland, who was born in 1905, practised as a Queen's Nurse on the islands of Fetlar in Shetland, Raasay, off the west coast of Scotland and back to Unst, Shetland. She followed in the foorsteps of her grannie, Mam Willa, who was a howdie. Mima now lives in Unst.

I did midwifery in Aberdeen Maternity Hospital in 1931 which was near Gordon Barracks. We had to pay to train. My sister trained in Elsie's and had to pay about ten pounds more than I did.

Some of the homes were very poor. One woman had nothing but a pile of *Radio Times* and the wifie downstairs gave me some clothes for the baby.

Aberdeen was a teaching hospital and we competed with students for cases. We often took them out with us on cases. They sometimes came from abroad. Usually a midwife there supervised the student and also had to subsidise the student's bus fares. They didn't have a maek. After midwifery training I went to Edinburgh to train for the Queen's Nursing certificate.

I got a post as a midwife in Fetlar where I did everything. I sat with an old lady every third night. When there was snow I had to walk four miles to the other side of the island. The taxi man used to walk with me and we wore stockings over our boots to walk in the snow. We walked arm in arm but when we came to the door we had to part company. I had to go in the 'professional' door and he, by the 'tradesman's entrance'. He would put his arms round me and give me a hug and say, 'You go in the proper door'. It was such a lonely place – Brough Lodge.

Scottish Midwives

Someone having a baby took priority. Someone would come and get me and then we had to walk. The doctor was Dr.Taylor, a contempory of Dr. Saxby. Wonderful man – a knight of the order of first class.

Often men and women never married. Mother said, 'I cannot understand it. This is a hippit generation'. But they were partners for life and there was no promiscuity. But the funny thing was very few had any results. There were not many births. We did the last offices too.

Next I went to the Island of Raasay in 1937. My friend was leaving and said I should apply for it. It was a lovely place full of trees and I stayed there till beginning of the war.

Raasay is not a fertile island. My sister was on the Island of Lismore then, off Oban – what a difference! There was such poor soil and it was very hard going on the little crofts there. Sometimes I had to go by boat to the beautiful little island of Fladda near Raasay, with four houses with a school mistress. Fishing was almost the only employment. I walked a lot in Raasay. We got a car from the garage to go the nine miles to the north end but if we were going on to Fladda you had to walk the additional five miles.

One 21st of June, I was called to Fladda. It was a terrible day for midsummer. The garageman put me the nine miles then I had to start walking. I ran down all the hills and pottered along and toiled up the next hill. It was about five miles to the shore and you could see the banks on the opposite side. If the tide was in, the boatman came across but if the tide was out you could walk across. On that day the baby had been born before I arrived and it was just wrapped up and I did the rest. I had to stay three days that time – in the same room as the patient. The beds had lovely fresh chaff on them.

Very soon, if the mother was well enough they had a function. I wish I could remember the Gaelic name for this ritual (see Chapter 8). All the women folk were invited and the father gave them a party. Everyone went upstairs and visited the mother still in bed. They brought presents for the baby and the midwife was there too. I would leave laden with presents – homemade jam and the like. They always had new head gear. I remember one time a girl came with a bargain book, a catalogue, to choose what to wear. In the old days the women all got new mutches for this party.

The woods on Raasay were owned by the Board of Agriculture and they let the people have firewood. The wifes carried big creels full of branches. At the back of each house the standard equipment was a double-ended saw which could be heard the whole time. The poor wifes wrocht hard carrying great creels full of branches. However, everybody accepted their lot. When they were having their babies they were fine but could have done with a lot more. When the war started it was awfully difficult to get butcher meat – maybe a pound of mince from the mainland. Everybody did their best but it was a lot poorer than Shetland.

The people were happy and the churches were active. They had a different outlook with Communions and Prayer Meetings. They never interfered with us but we fell into their ways, like not going for a walk on Sundays. They were a lovely people.

Then my father was asked to go to Unst – he was a policeman and the RAF Garrison was there. That was in 1939 just at the beginning of the war. He was very busy with wrecks coming ashore and people from Norway coming and waiting for transport. Dad just had a cycle and there were no police stations.

My parents were getting old and when the nurse on Unst left I got the job. It was wonderful coming home. All I wanted was to get back. There was no nurse's house on Unst and I lived with Dad and Mam. The Unst and Fetlar midwives stood in for each other.

In my time the mothers were all supervised antenatally. I saw them regularly and could test their urine. I would know if they needed to see the doctor. Later, you would wait for them to send for you. I cycled a lot and sometimes my father cycled with me. The airforce station was at Scaw and we cycled to Scaw to see a mother in a crofter's house which was inside the RAF station.

Later, we had a baby at the station. The clerk of works, an

English man and his wife – a very nice couple – had a wooden house in the centre of the Air Force camp. I had the supervision of her – she was a lovely lass and she was so brave. There were a lot of hit and run air raids here. One time we saw a plane coming. He gaed aroun and then we saw him coming again and Dad went to get his gun which he kept in a certain place. He went out but we pulled him inside and just not too soon. The plane came up from the south and in front of the door there were tracer bullets and two holes in the back of the hall. A woman was hurt and I had to go to her. She was in her door, looking. She got multiple injuries – I don't think she was ever the same again.

The station had some narrow escapes. When doctor and I went to this lady we had to wait at the gate before we were allowed in because there was an air-raid warning. By that time her husband had gone out on air-raid duty. She was awfully brave, the lass. She made supper and then doctor whispered to me, 'I don't think she'll be long now . I'll watch her while you have your supper'. As soon as supper was by she said to her friend, 'Mrs. Clarke, you'll need to wash the dishes. You'll need to excuse me'. She went to her room and the baby was born almost immediately.

I attended births myself very often but if I was worried about anything Dr Saxby would come with me. When we were together he would deliver the baby – you see he was a marvellous obstetrician – oh he was gifted. I would act as his assistant. He was renowned. My mother used to say it didn't matter whether Dr Saxby came to you in the middle of the day or the middle of the night, his linen was immaculate all the time.

Most times I went by myself. The mothers had everything ready. They would get in the wool. We used to get a reel of special ties for the umbilical cord.

My dad called me a peerie howdie. When I returned from a case he would be walking up and down and all he would say was, 'Is the woman all right?' and I would say, 'Yes she's fine'.

After the birth I used to see them twice a day. We were

supposed to see them 14 days. By the time they put their legs oot ower the side of the bed they would say, 'Look at my legs. What are they like?' They were wasted you see.

There was not a lot of breastfeeding. On to the bottle. They used one of the well-known powdered milks and National Dried and the orange juice. You did get some mothers who breastfed but a lot of mothers didn't seem to be able to do it.

One day I had twins. The second one was a breech. They were quite good weights – about six pounds. They knew they were having twins. A neighbour came in to help – there was always someone who would help. They're still here. One of them is a part-owner of the garage at Baltasound. He visits me every Christmas with a dram and always says, 'I can't think how you managed it'.

I think I was midwife on Unst for about twenty-six years. After I retired I took a degree from the Open University and I went to Stirling University for Summer School.

There was so much fun and people were so grateful. You get very close to the people being a midwife. It's very intimate especially when you think you are the person at the birth and the first person to see a new baby.

3

MARGARET FOGGIE

Margaret Foggie was born in South Africa in October 1908.
She came to Scotland in 1934 for the first time, to do
midwifery training. After qualifying as a midwife, Margaret
joined the Colonial Nursing Service and was sent initially to
Cyprus, where she met her husband. She now lives in Kirk-
caldy.

I'm South African and trained as a nurse in South Africa. I
came to London to do tropical diseases and when I passed the
finals I came to Rotten Row. I had never been in Scotland
before.

It was very hard work. We had lectures in our off duty. The
Sister Tutor read very quickly and you had to write out the
lectures neatly in your next off duty. We worked for the
whole six months. I started in summer 1934 and suddenly
realised when the summer was over that I had hardly seen a
green tree.

We wore a white uniform with collar and cuffs and on the
district a navy blue coat. We had little blue caps with white
strap round our chin and a bow at our throats, pinned on to
the hat with a bit of velvet – rather like the caps the Salvation
Army women wear.

Rottenrow is in the centre of Glasgow and at the time the
streets round about were very poor. The hospital was beau-
tifully kept, spartan, but very clean. I had great trouble
understanding the wifies, and the nurses too, because they
spoke with a strong Glasgow accent and used words which I
had never heard before. Like people 'going for their messages'. If something needed to be seen to, like the blind pulled
down, the blind needed 'sorted'. And – 'the barrows'. Some-

body told me to 'run down in the hoist to the second floor and bring up a barrow'. I realised the hoist was the lift, rushed down and couldn't see a barrow anywhere, only a few theatre trolleys. I returned and said I could only find a few theatre trolleys. She said, 'But that's what I want!' Another phrase was, 'weans were greeting [children were crying]'. It was a whole new language.

A lot of mothers with quite normal pregnancies came in for delivery. However, any mothers with an abnormality from the West of Scotland and the Islands came to us. If we were full we sent them to Stobhill. I was awfully lucky. I had a month in the theatre in my six months so I saw Caesareans and all sorts of odd operations and abnormalities. I enjoyed theatre work.

The training was very interesting but terribly hard work. On night duty on our day off for the month, we could get up at eleven a.m. but we had to be back by eleven p.m. We had no pay at all. Parents helped out. My stepmother sent me money every month. You could exist because they fed you but that was all.

There was a famous old Matron there – she was a very fierce old thing. She snooped round at night and always found something wrong. Even the sisters used to cringe. But the place on the whole was quite well run.

During our six months' training we were out on district for a month. We didn't live in the hospital then. There was a special building where the people on district lived because they felt they got their clothes contaminated. We always took newspaper with us because it was cleaner than the sheets or whatever they had on the beds. There were bugs and various things on the walls. I don't remember fleas or being bitten but I never knew where to hang my coat in the houses. I would wrap it up in some of the newspaper. It was used for everything.

Very few of the men were working. The *Queen Mary* was up on the stocks. Unemployment was terrible and there was such a kind of despair about it. It was a very bad time. Glasgow Corporation produced a layette for the new baby if the woman went to the antenatal clinic and got a form saying she was pregnant. Very often they didn't even bother to go and collect it and there was nowhere to put the baby except a drawer if you could find one. There was such a feeling of apathy. Even in some of the new tenements which had baths they didn't use them. I actually have seen coal in the bath. I had never seen people living like that. It was wonderful to think of the new birth and a dear little baby – but the people were very dispirited and it was quite dispiriting for us too.

My first night on the district I went to a house where the woman had never been to the antenatal clinic and she had eclampsia and epilepsy. We had special notepads and if you had a problem you wrote a message which someone took to the police. They contacted the hospital by phone and a doctor would come out. So on this occasion I sent my message and the doctor came.

In the beginning you went out by yourself with your black bag and phoned in to say how you were getting on. We had been in hospital for four or five months. As students we went out all alone while the medical students always went in twos. The police went in sixes. As far as I know nothing ever happened.

Once we were out with someone in labour, we stayed and delivered the baby, with back-up if you were worried. It was quite a responsibility. I don't think they realised we were not qualified. They just accepted that the 'nurse' came. We had to have twenty deliveries during the training and they all had to be properly written up in a special book.

We were taught in Rottenrow to bath the baby on our knee. They said we had to learn to do the babies on our knee because there was nowhere else to do it. Somebody in the close would boil some water for you and we took soap with us. We delivered the baby straight on to newspapers. There were these beds in the wall where they all slept and you had to turn father and all the children out whilst mother produced her thirteenth. There were huge families. Sometimes the father was still in the bed. If he was working during the day he had to have his sleep and the midwife would have to get him out at the last moment. I always managed to do that earlier to give me a clear run. The poor mothers didn't really want another baby after they had had nine or ten children.

The lectures were absolutely excellent. The Sister Tutor was very good and her notes were much better than the textbook. She was very clear about the head entering the pelvis and that sort of thing. Various doctors came and gave us lectures and they were excellent too. We had textbooks written by three doctors each in charge of a ward. The senior doctor was an old Doctor Cameron. He came from Dumfries and was in charge of the ground floor.

There were two long wards, one postnatal and the other prenatal. One night I was alone in prenatal when a woman said she wanted a bedpan. When I gave her it she produced a baby with no pains at all. It was extraordinary. I was quite new at that time. I had not been to the labour ward at this point and I didn't know what to do. However, I picked up the telephone and got the sister in charge and she came galloping along. Her first baby – and mine too!

On Sundays the weans were all fed early and taken away to the nursery. We drew down all the blinds and took away all the wifies' papers and women's magazines and hid them in the lockers and put a Bible on each bed. But the blinds were drawn so they couldn't read them anyhow. At 3.30pm the blinds were pulled up, the Bibles were collected, the wifies could put their papers back on the lockers and the weans were all greeting. This was the sop to Sunday.

I came across a lot of women with rickety pelves in Glasgow. They attributed this to the water which came from Loch Katrine and there was no lime in it at that time. A lot of people ware bandy-legged too.

Some of the places I went to were so poor and dirty and lacking in any sort of conveniences. They lived in one room with a bed in the wall and a communal lavatory. I don't know where their water was. They didn't have it in their room – what they called their house. It must have been on the stairs. When the new houses were built they had baths and running water. Some of the closes and tenements were awful. There was a place called Garngad which was worse than the Gorbals – slops in the street – very dirty. It was all so sad and pathetic. I had never seen people living in those sort of conditions. Things may have been bad in our slums in Johannesburg and other places in South Africa but nothing as bad as that.

The district office in the hospital had big maps of the area and they gave you instructions of where to go – take tram 37 to whatever street and so on. You also visited postnatally for some days to examine the mother and baby. Sometimes you had to see someone you hadn't delivered. You got about five or six houses to visit.

We had to try and keep the mothers in bed. This was very difficult and we couldn't insist on it. We would tell the husband to remember his wife was not well. 'Run the messages and look after the weans.' They would say yes, but very often I don't think they did it. They used to stand around on the street talking.

Whilst I was there they started on the *Queen Mary* again. It would have been the summer of 1934 and the bands played the workers on to the job. Some of the wifies' husbands were working and they were so superior and pleased. 'My man's working.'

When women were admitted to Rotten Row they were taken to what was called 'the slab'. I suppose it was to get rid of vermin. They undressed the women and hosed them down on this concrete slab before they were allowed further. It was awful to do that. They would then have a clean nightie put on. I don't think everybody who came in went through the slab.

Very often a mother would ask what your name was because they wanted to call the baby after you. By the time they had had ten babies it was difficult to find names. If they already had a Margaret, did I have another name? There was one woman who said, 'I'd like to call my baby Vagina. I think it's such a nice word'. I nearly had a fit. So I said, 'Why not call her Regina?' I don't know what she eventually did. She just liked the sound of the word.

They were very keen on breastfeeding at the hospital. Sometimes they did have to use artificial stuff. I think it was Glaxo. The mothers were told to breastfeed and before feeding time you had to run round and swab all their nipples so that they were nice and clean and then when they had finished feeding you swabbed them again. They all breast fed if possible. It mostly is possible but some people don't like it or don't want to. Mothers having a home birth all breast fed too. It was much easier for them.

I don't remember any mothers dying. If anyone was very ill in the wards they were taken to a special department and looked after there. The mothers I looked after in the hospital were all healthy. Any baby that was sickly received special treatment in the nursery. Otherwise the babies were all kept in the wards with their mothers in cots at the foot of the beds.

The food for the wifies – they used to get porridge in the morning. I don't remember what else they got. I don't think they got a lot of visiting. Husbands used to come but I don't remember hordes of people coming – not like nowadays. They were afraid of infection .

I got my hospital certificate there but I decided to take my CMB examination in London. You could do that then. There was a written part and a viva. I found the written paper quite easy and enjoyed the viva. It was held in a huge room. The examiners – two doctors, a man and a woman, not very old – sat at a table. They asked me a few questions about abnormalities of various sorts. Then they said, 'Is there anything that you would like to talk about?' There was a pelvis on the table and I said, 'Yes, I'd like to talk about abnormal pelves and disproportion'. They looked a bit nonplussed. They hardly got any of that in London. So I talked about trial of labours and heads entering the pelvis in the wrong place and so on. They sat open-mouthed as I told them about what I had experienced and how they did trial labours in Glasgow. Then I said, 'I think I've told you all I can tell you'. They seemed really interested and both, there and then, offered me jobs. However, I didn't really want to carry on with midwifery. I told them and thanked them very much. Who they were I don't know.

Sometimes the wifies were worried about the baby surviving and asked if you would christen the baby. Well, I'm an Episcopalian and a lot of the wifies were Roman Catholics. There was one woman who was in a terrible state wanting her baby christened and I knew she was a Roman Catholic so I said, 'You know I'm not a *Roman* Catholic but I am a Catholic because I believe in it'. So she said, 'Christen my baby'. She was in such a state that I christened the baby and she was happy. That's important. She wanted it for her baby. It's funny, I haven't thought of that for years.

4

CHRISSIE SANDISON

Since she was a small girl, Chrissie Sandison, of Aith in Shetland, has observed people. Her gifts of remembering and story-telling are well known locally. Here she recalls incidents and characters surrounding childbirth.

When I was a child in the 1920s the doctor was good and the women liked him but he would never fetch the midwife until she was required. With my aunt's second baby, she said he sat downstairs reading and never went upstairs until the midwife went to the lavatory a good bit from the house. It was a wee house across a burn. There was no bucket, just a seat across a burn and toilet roll was likely a bit of newspaper and no buckets to empty. When she had to go, the doctor went up to inspect how the mother was progressing and then when she came back he would go downstairs again.

When she had her next baby in 1929 she employed another woman who had a big family but wasn't a certified midwife. Then the doctor was quite happy. He didn't like working with the trained midwife. I think he thought she knew as much as he did.

Another woman I knew was not happy with the midwife she had for her first and ever after that she had – not a howdie – just a neighbour. In the early 1920s the women never had any examinations or care beforehand. I remember Jimmy's mother telling me about when she was young and having her children. It was kept a secret until she was sure and then she would speak to some old neighbour, somebody she knew would help, and they kept it a secret. So, an expectant mother *at da faain-fit* [getting near the time of delivery] would have 'spoken for' a midwife. You see they didn't do much – nature did it. A lot of midwifery is just waiting. Sometimes all went well, sometimes not – with tragic consequences.

Another woman, Betty Hall from Gonfirth, South Delting was often called upon. She did OK so long as nature was kind but one time in May 1933 she was unable to remove the placenta. The house was far from a road and no doctor near to call upon. The mother was in great danger until several hours later the doctor appeared and put things right. It was a close thing.

In another incident around 1930 a woman aged forty having her first baby, had a contracted pelvis. (I discovered this not long ago from coming across the registration of her death). I think Dr. Henry from Voe was fetched. The infant couldn't be born so the surgeon from Lerwick was summoned. I'm not sure whether an operation was done at the house or if the infant was taken away piecemeal. I was twelve at the time so these things were not discussed in my presence. Anyway the poor mother didn't survive. She died a day or two later.

I remember going to the house the next morning. They always had me for a go-between. I was to go and see how she was and take a bottle of milk as they didn't have any animals. We liked her very much. She was about 40 and this was her first baby. They explained to me that the baby was born and was dead. I mind yet there was a box standing up in the corner. I wondered if that's where the baby would be but I never asked anybody.

The next day I was sent again and the next. There was a midwife there that day because I met her. She was outside and the woman who was dead, she was also outside. It was April. When I went in the house a neighbour, a young woman, was there. There are always folk that go to people in distress. When I went in with the milk I never spoke. I didn't know what to say. She came across to me and said that Tilly had died. I never cried but I was very upset. It was maybe shock. I went home to my aunt and my sister. I don't know why they sent me I'm quite sure that woman had no pre-natal examinations.

Chrissie Sandison

Premature babies were kept at home and not washed. They rubbed them with goose grease and wrapped them up in sheep's wool and took turns to sit by the fire with the baby to keep it warm. There was another very small baby where the mother died. Four or six weeks after the birth the baby took whooping-cough from his brothers and sisters. He was kept by the fire in a cradle and the women took turns to sit with him – they had their knitting – and every time that child began to cough they got him up. If ever anybody was in any kind of trouble, the neighbours rallied around. That baby lived. They also used goose grease during the birth of a baby, or a cow calving. Maybe that was what is now referred to as 'Back to basics!'

Unmarried women sadly didn't get much attention. They had blotted their copybook. One time, a woman's mother knew she was going to have a baby but pretended she didn't. This woman was in her thirties and she already had one ten-year- old. One day she went into labour and somebody going past noticed her acting strangely outside. The postman saw what was going on when he came in for his cup of tea. She went into the yard amongst the corn and they began to think things were happening. The old mother got her inside, pushed her up the stair, threw some clothes up after her and then got the midwife. The baby was born right enough and in the evening the old woman at the well said, 'Well you never know in the morning what you're going to be saying at night'. Everybody else knew what was on the go. Everybody wasn't like that. Some just accepted them and the baby was just swallowed up in the family with the other bairns.

Multiple birth

Triplets were born at home on 26 August 1927. The mother, K., was thirty-seven and was staying with her mother, at Vird – a small thatch-roofed house right at the innermost reaches of East Burrafirth Voe. Also in the house were her brother, Jamie and her niece, W. who was eight. Her husband was away at the fishing.

In the middle of the night K. went into labour. She was sharing the ben-end sleeping quarters with her mother who had seven children herself. She roused both J. and W. J. had to go for Dr. Bowie who lived at Parkhall – west past Bixter – and W. was given a howling infant to hold. Then her grandmother shouted, 'My God, here's another one!' She laid number one wrapped in an old petticoat into the basket chair and was handed the second squalling infant.

In the meantime, J. had made himself a cup of tea while his mother urged him to hurry. She had no idea there might be another one.

J. had a mile or more to run to get someone to row him across the voe. Then he hired a car to Parkhall to get the doctor and take him back to East Burrafirth. When he eventually roused the doctor he said, 'Our K. is having some children! There's one in the basket chair, and one on the lid of the kist and God knows how many more!'

When Dr. Bowie arrived he discovered there was still an infant waiting to be born. It was a boy – stillborn. Doctor said if he had been there twenty minutes earlier he might have saved him but if he had been twenty minutes later the mother would have been gone.

I don't think a midwife was there afterwards. I think a local woman went along in the morning to wash and feed the two peerie girls. Only one survived – the other one died aged four weeks. That was a very humble dwelling even by the standards of that time when folk were pretty ignorant about lots of things yet it's marvellous how well they managed. There was no running water except the burn flowing past, just an open fireplace, and the but and ben. Primitive conditions.

All that makes one think of the vast changes even within my eighty years' lifespan. Nowadays that mother would be airlifted to Aberdeen. I can well understand how a shroud would be laid in the kist once a young woman got married. Quite a few women died during or after childbirth. I marvel that so many survived and had maybe fourteen or more children. A stillbirth was accepted as God's will and soon the mother was pregnant again. My own mother gave birth to

Chrissie Sandison

ten including two stillbirths. I was the youngest. She died of
kidney failure aged forty-six when I was aged one year and
nine months.

Baby clothes

Many winter babies in Shetland didn't get outside until the
spring. 'Never let them see outside.' First they had a binder
round the umbilicus.The first ones I mind were flannelette.
Then a sort of elastic bandage was used. I think they gave it
two turns and then sewed it on. Then they had a winter thing,
a winceyette barry-coat, sleeveless and all tapes, and you
could open it to change the baby's nappy. It was long enough
to cover the feet. Then, a long cotton frock, perhaps something thicker in winter. When I was going round looking at
babies I mind seeing they had the frock turned up around the
baby's head. I think it was to stop it getting wet. No plastic
pants.

Folk had no money. I mind one family with a few children.
They had a creel and a flour bag from the shop. This
probably held seventy pounds of flour, was bleached white
and stuffed with straw. It was soft Shetland oats so it wasn't
stiff like Scots oats. That was the bed and the pillow was
something soft like wool inside a small pillow case. Another
thing I mind was in one house where they were not very well
off, a grey or fawn woman's underskirt cut up and spread out
for a blanket. Before the baby was laid in it, it was warmed
before the fire and sometimes it had a strong smell. The baby
was fine and cosy and then they rocked the baby to sleep.
They then would have a quilt made out of old bits and pieces.

When a mother was having a baby they got a bar of Pears
Soap exclusively to bath the baby.They never had toilet soap
at any other time.It had the same smell then as now. They
bathed the baby every night. When a couple got married
someone always gave them a couple of pairs of white towels
to spread out when they bathed the baby. But I just wonder
how some folk managed.

33

Feeding

They nearly all breast fed unless a mother died. I don't think I was breastfed as my mother was forty-four when she had me. My aunt said I was so small they didn't know if I was going to survive. We had a calved cow – calved in September and I was born in the November. They thought her milk would be too strong for me so they put me on a farrow cow that had calved some time and the milk likely wasn't so strong. I think the bottles I remember from the 1930s are yon ones wi the tube. To clean it, the mother put it in soapy water, put the tube into her mouth and breathed in and out. They couldn't boil the rubber. Dr Hunter told me not so long ago, about a woman boasting to him that's how she fed all her children. She had seven or eight. It was very dangerous as they used to go out and leave the child alone with it and the child could choke. They just put the bottle alongside the cot and put the teat in its mouth. They wouldn't get wind as the glass bit went right down to the bottom of the bottle.

Weaning

I don't think they were very old before they got bits off a spoon. They used to steep oatmeal overnight and then boil the juice off it. It was called oatmeal water. There was also MOF and Sister Laura's food. There was another kind of stuff called Slippery Elm and fish in milk. Also wet nursing. A mother who didn't have much milk went to another who had a lot and one fed the other's baby. Also, if a mother had engorged breasts and no breast pump, to relieve them someone just sucked off the milk.

There was another time when a cyclist was seeing someone in Lerwick and she was in agony with engorged breasts and he offered to suck it off. They say he got home to North Mavine in record time. I couldn't imagine it because when I remember him he was an old man wi a mouser. They had no other way of doing it. It's very painful and that was common practice. There was a lot more helping. Everybody helped each other.

5

MOLLY MUIR

Molly Muir was born in 1907 and did her midwifery training in the 'Old Simpson' in Edinburgh in 1934. She worked as a private nurse and midwife in many places in Scotland. Latterly, Molly lived in Edinburgh. She died in early 2000.

I trained in the old Simpson in 1934 from June until December and thirty of us sat the written and oral exam in the Royal College of Surgeons in February 1935. On the same day we heard we had all passed. Many of these girls came up from London because of the difference in price between the top London hospitals and here. It was £45 for Simpson's and £62 for Queen Charlotte's. I would have quite liked to have gone to Queen Charlotte's but I wanted to practise with the doctors I knew and also money was a consideration. We weren't paid at that time. We didn't have to buy our uniform but it wasn't supplied either. We could wear our uniform from our general training so there were all sorts of uniforms from different hospitals.

After finishing general training and becoming a fourth-year nurse you came down to earth with a bump starting at Simpson's as a pupil midwife. Something I found terribly difficult to start with was finding the fetal heart. I had quite a job and I remember being quite excited when I heard the first one with a Pinard's stethoscope.

There were only three wards in the old Simpson's so you got to know everybody. The labour ward had seven beds with Sister Anderson, who was also the sister of the district, in charge. She was very good and looked after us all very well. Miss Ferlie was the matron and she moved to the new Simpson in the early years of the war. I liked working in labour ward best but as a student midwife you did everything. A bedpan round was a tremendous business. Now they don't have such a thing. Patients get up just after the baby is born.

I think a nurse from Barts and I held the record for quick baby-bathing. We had to examine the babies from top to toe. The cord had to be dressed with a binder which was stitched on, every day. When the baby was ready we took it to the mother and sometimes you had quite a bit of difficulty getting the baby feeding. The mothers took it for granted they would breastfeed unless something went wrong. Then, we took the milk off with a pump, put it in a bottle and the baby would get breastmilk that way.

No-one was off in the morning because all the babies had to be bathed, the mothers attended to and the bedpan round and swabbings. We went to the medical part of the university for our lectures and it was pandemonium getting ready for that because everything had to be done on the ward before we went away. We went running up Lady Lawson Street on our way to the Royal, getting on our coats and hats. Sister would be alone in the ward while we were away. The lectures lasted about an hour and we ran back. There would be another bedpan round then.

We started at 8 a.m. and worked until 8 p.m. with three hours off in the middle and one half-day per week. No days off. On Sundays we came on duty in the morning and finished at 1 p.m. and the other crowd came on then for the rest of the day and we changed each weekend.

Night duty was busy. We had to keep the crying babies quiet because the mothers had to get their sleep. Babies were in cots beside the mother's bed. If the baby cried we lifted it and quietened it. There was never a break.

Our rooms took about six but we were so tired we could sleep anywhere. It wasn't in the hospital. It was up the road beside the Fire Station and that was noisy but it didn't matter. If you were on district for the outside cases you could be called out, it didn't matter where. Most nights someone was called out – we took it in turns. When we were on call we could be called out three times in a week and were expected to do our normal work during the day after this. We never had a qualified midwife with us as we were nearly at the end of our training.

I walked every morning from the old Simpson's to Gorgie which was my district. There, I bathed my babies and dealt with the mothers for about two weeks postnatally. Most of them had a good neighbour who helped who we always called Maggie and who was there the whole time, in the background, making tea and scones and supplying hot water to bath the baby as there was no hot water in the tap. The neighbours like Maggie were the nicest people and very important. They were so excited when the baby was born.

One time I did the mother and bathed the baby and then I said, 'You know you've got on awfully well. I think you could get up this afternoon for an hour'. I carried on further up the street to another lady and she said, 'Hasn't Mrs S. done well. She was up having tea with me yesterday afternoon'. So you never knew what was happening when your back was turned. They weren't ill. She was pretending that she was doing all that she was supposed to be doing.

During the night we always had a medical student with us. We usually did the delivery as I think they were just beginning that part of their training. We weren't allowed to walk alone at night although I'm quite sure in uniform we would have been quite safe. There weren't many police out at night. We didn't use tramcars because it was too roundabout a route from Simpson's to Gorgie by tram so we just walked. Anyway we wouldn't have had a penny for the fare. Once I had an Egyptian student with me going out to a case. He was a very nice man and seemed to have any amount of money and wanted to take a taxi as he wasn't used to walking. I said we wouldn't have a taxi and made him walk.

There were very few antenatal clinics but when a woman was pregnant and knew she had to book a midwife for the delivery, it was arranged quite far in advance. When the time came we would be notified from a public telephone.

Because there was very little antenatal care, sometimes we were taken by surprise when the mother was in labour. The worst I had was a face presentation. There were very few deaths of mothers – there was only the one that I knew of. She died and the baby died. We had just the odd stillbirth but not a great many. I never had a death outside on the district.

You can understand why they wanted to have their babies at home when they had other children. Also, they would be up the next day, unofficially, instead of being in bed for two weeks. The amount of DVT was the beginning of getting them out of their beds earlier. Homes all had fathers and many of the fathers were very good at looking after the children – not all of them but most of them. There was a lot of unemployment. One night I went to a case in the High Street, a thirteenth child. They had one room with two double beds where they all slept and the father was unemployed. While I was dealing with the birth the father got the others up and took them out to walk the streets. I don't know why they didn't have neighbours in to help. That was in the High Street when the High Street houses were really slums.

That night the student with me was spotless. He had on a lovely forget-me-not blue shirt just stiff with being well washed and ironed. A great fat bug jumped on to his sleeve which I took with my fingers, threw on the floor and stood on. Apart from that we had a lot of lice and fleas. We didn't have to delouse ourselves because we wore caps closely on our heads and the whole idea of the cap was to keep the lice from your hair and so keep your hair clean. Now, they put a piece of ribbon or a piece of lace on their heads and that's supposed to be a cap. It's no good at all.

I always remember that night. No blankets on the bed, just covered with old coats. We took a rubber draw sheet to put under the mother to deliver the baby and in this house they only had one chair. I bathed the baby in a baking bowl, and the next morning I went back with clothes for the baby. At Simpson's we were given clothes from people who were finished with them. We could always draw on that. This mother didn't have a cot for the baby. He stayed in bed with the mother, and probably another half-dozen children climbed in as well. That was her thirteenth, the most I ever came across, and I don't know if that was her last child or not. By the 1930s people were beginning to talk about family planning but many didn't use anything. They had very big families.

One night a medical student and I went out to a very nice house in Gorgie. The woman was a long time in labour.We went out just after midnight and came in after 8 a.m. At Simpson's, breakfast was at 8 a.m. and if you weren't there, you didn't get any. The student suggested we should have a cup of coffee at Tollcross before we went in but I said no, because the mother we had delivered might phone in with a problem and Sister Anderson wouldn't know where we were. When we arrived, Sister Anderson said there was a nice big parcel for me. This turned out to be a food parcel from my mother so I asked Sister if we could go and have coffee before starting the district. The student was coming with me – to help, even though he wasn't supposed to. We took this parcel containing a piece of roast lamb and homemade scones and butter and with 4/6 between us we could afford a *pot* of coffee not just a cup. We had a right feast.

We were always short of money. We had everything else but money.and although I got parcels to augment the very poor food, I didn't expect to get money from home. One girl's father was a wealthy farmer somewhere up north and she would say to me, 'Can you give me a penny, I've got nothing less than a pound' and I never had a pound. The thought of giving me back a penny would never enter her head.

When we went to Princes Street we were always properly dressed including a hat. We used to go dancing which I loved, to the Fountainhall Palais some nights when we were off in the evening, maybe out with a student who had more money. We were very happy.

When I finished I did private nursing. In these days if you were a sister in a hospital, the salary was eighty pounds a year whether you had been there two years or twenty years. In private nursing if it was a baby case it was four guineas a week although if you weren't working you weren't paid. I did a whole year of baby cases with no day off because the cases ran into each other. I was acting as a monthly nurse and you would probably go to the case a week before labour started, which put you all wrong for your next case. It was very hard work but I loved it. I loved looking after those babies. I did the postnatal care of the mothers as well. I used to go to places like Saline, North Berwick, Berwick-on-Tweed, Carlisle – wherever they wanted a midwife. We had our headquarters in Rutland Street with Miss Drummond as matron and there were about eighty trained nurses/midwives on the staff going out to different cases.

I only once had to call a doctor when I was on my baby cases after I was trained. This mother was in her late thirties, having her first baby and having a very difficult time. We called the doctor who came and delivered the baby. I'm quite sure that today she would have had a Caesarean section but there were very few done then. She had a forceps delivery with a very bad pelvic floor tear and no pain relief.

In the Simpson's I worked with a midwife who was so good and kind, and slow and gentle in all her movements. I thought, that is the way to deliver babies. The slower the better to help the mother, and everything so gentle and quiet.

6

ANNIE KERR

Annie Kerr was born in November 1900. She had her own babies before she started caring for mothers as an uncertified midwife in the countryside around Castle Douglas during the Second World War.

When my husband died I had to work. I went oot as a midwife. I got on to it through the doctor. My own doctor, Doctor Ford, was away at the war and we had to go to Dr Welsh. He knew I likit these jobs away oot the road of everybody and no other body would go near them because – I can min a young woman sayin to me, 'Oh, gaan there? Ye wouldna get back hame til Christmas.' They wouldna hae naethin tae dae wi it. Aa the housework, and the lady forbye, wi the baby. I went a wee while before the baby wis born. I wis with them and did everything that wis to be done to give her a rest.

Dr Welsh gied me great jobs. He'd be attendin her an watchin her aa the time and he would know when the baby wis due. He aye got there in time. I had nocht tae dae wi sendin for the doctor. Her ain man wid send. I was there when the baby came. It didna bother me in the least. I wisna daein the gruntin! Mines wis aa bye by then.

I didna deliver the baby myself. It was always the doctor. My mother had neither doctor nor onybody. She cut the cord and tied it. She must hae been a strong woman. I couldna hae daen that.

I would gie the baby its first bath and I took care of the baby afterwards until the mother wis fit. I wid mebbe be there a fortnight. It wis reckoned they shouldna be out o bed till the nine days were up. That wis quite common. Ye weren't

41

allowed up but I remember one woman gettin up. The baby began to cry and I took no notice of it. I got on with the bakin in the kitchen and when I came in, here she was sittin wi the baby. She had got up and walked across to the baby, and picked it up. I got sic a shock when I saw her. She was never any the worse of it. They liked to get ye up on yer feet. It saved clottin.

I canna min how lang I did it. I went tae a wheen houses and met an affae lot o folk, nice folk. I made a lot o friends. If I had time I used to go back and visit them.

When I was stayin with the women havin their babies I did everything. The washing, cleaning, into Castle Douglas for the messages. On the big farm they had what we caa'ed a lass and they worked helpin in the hoose, and there wid mebbe be twae young men forbye. That made three extra folk in the house to bake for. So I had all that to look after. The mother would see to hersel by that time if she was fit. I took care of her when she was in bed. I didna let her work while I was there. That's what I was there to dae – to work and save her till she gathered her own strength again. I gave her a basin to wash herself. I never took nowt tae dae wi the washin. I looked after the baby and everything for her and did aa the housework. I was busy but I enjoyed it. Dr Ford didn't give a damn what ye were daein but Dr Welsh was the very opposite. He attended and looked after ye. I liked him, Dr Welsh. He was a nice man.

There were nurses and they aa went on bikes. I think the nurse would come just the same. She would have to come and look after the mother. When it was away up in the hills it was just me. Nurse MacDougal was the nurse and the midwife then. She gied me a lot o jobs. She stopped working when she got married.

The mothers and babies were aa fine. If they werena we would ha had the doctor. I could only stay with them so long because I was booked away in front. So I had to go from one to the other. I didna get much rest.

I got paid. I wouldna dae it for nocht. I think I got about two pounds or fifty bob a week. That was a lot in thae days. I charged the same wherever I went. And my keep. I thought I was quite well off and I enjoyed it. I likit the babies aa right. They likit their splash. The baby used to lie on my hand in the bath and I could splash the wee one. Oh aye, they did enjoy it. On their knees and they could loup.

I helped with the breastfeeding. Ye had to watch that they got their nipples cleaned for the babies. I helped them put the baby to the breast. I did everything for them that I could dae. I've had babies wi bottles – everything.

The cord – that was their navel. That was cut. I would tie it and then I cut it. I put a binder on it and I also put a penny on the navel to keep it in. I expect not having the doctor there when the baby was born it wouldna be richt looked efter. I think a doctor should ha been there. Bit they aa lived. I wouldna ha liked to be on my own. I was always sittin waitin. The doctor was aye there sittin waitin. He would never touch the baby or the mother until she was fully – what – dilated, it was a word like that. He wouldn't touch them until a certain time. He sat and waited and talked to the mother in the kitchen and I wondered how long he was going to wait? I would have got fed up waitin. But he wouldn't touch the mother until they were fully dilated.

They didn't get chloroform wi me. Not with the doctor either, no while I was there. I had chloroform with one of my babies and it made me sick and I told the doctor I wasn't having any of that damned stuff any more.

They had lots o babies. There was aye time for that. They would want me back because it's no everyone that would dae the work and look after the mother. The midwives would only look after the mother and baby. They wouldna dae housework. This is why mebbe they wanted me.

Wee June, my youngest, sometimes came wi me, sometimes not. Sometimes she stayed wi Betty. I was working on this big farm where there were two brothers and I told Mrs Mac-Adam I was going into Castle Douglas to meet Betty and she was bringin wee June. I can min on meetin them in Castle Douglas and that's what brought me home. I'll never forget June. She just stared at me. Betty came off the bus and met me at Castle Douglas at this park. She had wee June in her arms. And wee June just looked at me and never moved. That put me right off goin out. I never went out again. I just said to myself, well my ain dashed weans disna ken me. So that finished that. I got that many letters wanting me. I had to tell them that I wisna goin out ony longer.

It was quite good fun. I enjoyed it.

7

DODDIE DAVIDSON

Doddie Davidson worked in the 1930s and '40s in the North-East of Scotland looking after mothers in labour, delivering their babies and caring for them afterwards. As well as this, she kept house, looked after the other children and cooked meals for the family and anyone else who happened to be there. She was known as 'the howdie'.

I wis jist aboot eighteen when I delivered ma first baby. That wis Babs. Her mother asked me if I wid look efter Babs at the time and I said, 'Oh, aye, I would try'. I'd never seen a bairn bein born afore. Fan she went inti labour, she said, ' I've usually plenty time. There's nothing to worry aboot'. She'd hid twa babies afore that. But in the evenin it came on sna an the pains real strong and quick an I gid oot fur her hubby. It wis a fairm awa on its own like. I said, 'Ye'd better ging fur the doctor', an he set aff afore it got ower bad. Ye didna tell the doctor aforehand. He jist cam fan ye needed them. This wis at Moss Farm, Slains.

By the time he got tae Hatton it wis blin drift and the roads were blockit an the peer doctor hid tae walk fae Hatton back tae this fairm and walk back again. It would ha been aboot five mile. Meantime Babby wis gettin on wi't an I thocht, ' Oh I'd better get tools an things ready'. Ah kent foo tae dae at. So I got tools an bilin watter for the doctor comin. Twa oors later I could see the baby's heid comin. There wis naebiddy here but me. There wisna neighbours ye see. So I thocht, 'Fit'll I dae?' I said, 'It winna be lang noo Babby'. But the heid jist didna come ony further. I thocht, 'At baby disna look richt tae me. I na ken fit tae dae'. I could see there wis twa cords on its neck. The heid wis oot an it didna look richt. It

45

wis jist growin bluer. I said, 'Babs, I'm nae sure, I'll maybe hurt ye but I'm daein ma best, ye ken'. She wis in pain bit she wisna bothered as lang as I did something. I pushed the heidie back a wee bittie and I got one finger in below the cord and I got it ower – the second bit o the cord wis easy, it wis the first at wis afa ticht. Efter I got at daen, the baby wis born, nae doctor, nae hubby, naebiddy. I hid tae wrap it – bit the baby wis motionless, an blue. An I thocht, 'It's deid'. But I wrappit it up wi a tool an – the cord wisna cut or naethin. It sort a gid a kin a half-cough and then anither cough, sort a spluttered a bittie and I thocht, 'Well it's still here'. Aa at eence it gid a yell and I wis never so pleased to hear a bairn. Nae only at, I wis scared I'd daen wrang pittin the baby back a bit. There wis nae wey else I could ha got the cord aff.

A while efter at, the doctor an her hubby came back an he looked at the baby an he said, 'Fit, is this been corded?' The marks wis still on the neck. I said, 'Aye', an I telt him. I wis fair shakkin wi fit I did. So he commended me. He said, 'Oh at wis jist great. I could dae wi you on the district'. It wis OK. I wis wi him a few times efter at.

Ye nivver forget on at because it wis a bad stairt an tae nae hae ony nursin experience . Some folk would ha jist left it but I think sometimes common sense helps a bittie. I did one or two mair jobs for him afore we moved awa tae Barthol Chapel. I wisna so worried again.

I gaed tae onybiddy that wis needin, but I wid aye mak sure the doctor came. Sometimes they kent there wis a baby expectit, sometimes they didna. This wis in the thirties. They hid nae antenatal care. He wid ken aboot a baby comin if the mother hid been ill or if some of the bairns hid been bad an he'd been up tae the hoose. Bit itherwise they didna get ony lookin efter.

I lived in the hoose afore the bairns were born. There wis naebiddy there bit me. Sometimes, if there wis a neighbour handy she wid come in, bit fairms is usually on their ain an it wis maistly cotter hooses or fairms. It wis aa fowk at mebbe wisna weel aff. The weel aff fowk could aford mebbe somebody better. There wis nae midwife. They ca'ed ye the howdie. Fan ye arrived they said, 'Are you the howdie?' I aye kent in time afore. Usually they were needin some help especially fan there wis some little eens. Then ye stayed, sometimes a wik sometimes mair, sometimes ye didna hae time tae spare but ye aye hid aboot a wik wi them or ten days. I did quite a lot, some o the names I canna even min.

I hid Mrs McA. but she hid twins an triplets afore my time. Fan I wis there it wis triplets again but the doctor didna ken she wis pregnant and she lost twa o them. Een wis stillborn. They werena taen intil the hospital like now. They jist lived or died an that wis it. Jist a young lassie, I think she wis aboot twenty-four. She hid an afa hanfae. The wee loon he wis jist aboot three pounds. I jist wrappit him in nappies. In those days ye hid muslin nappies an toolin nappies. I pit a muslin nappy roon him and then a toolin een. Ye couldna dress him, he wis that little. He wis in aside his Mam tae keep him warm. The babies werna putten in cots the same. An ye nivver heard o a cot death either. I often wunner aboot them bein taen awa fae their mithers sae quick. There wis thirteen o us and aye in the first year the bairn wis in wi ma mither. Aa hame births every one.

We spoon fed that wee loonie. Jist drops. We took aff his Mam's milk. Ye didna need much. But he lived, which wis a great thing. I wis aboot three wiks we her, a good whilie. Ye could see the baby wis growin – he wis an afa wee pop. But noo he wid be straight intil an incubator. She hid aa that ither babies an they aa lived.

Folk began to send for me from different places – Slains, Newmachar, Stoneywood. There were two at Stoneywood. They were neighbours and there wis six wiks atween their dates. Een wis aboot three wiks late, that wis Mrs L, and then fan her baby wis born she gaed intae fits. Her man gaed awa fur the doctor again an she wis taen intil the hospital, and the baby. But she had the three ither eens at hame an Ah wis tae be wi her next-door neighbour six wiks efter Mrs L. This wis a kinna late baby fur her. She cam in tae see fit wis goin on wi an ambulance at the door. She gid intil sic a state *her* baby started tae arrive three wiks early.

I promised Mrs L I wid stay wi the bairns or she got oot o the hospital. I kent that the next door ane wis needin me onywey. She hid two as weel, two little anes. Mrs L's bairns wis up a bit. The other woman's baby wis born at night. The peer doctor hid tae come back again. We hidna lang tae wait. I delivered it. It wis aboot six pounds. Mrs L, the een that took the fits, her baby wis big, aboot eight pounds. She wis OK efter. She wis in the hospital wi the baby aboot ten days. The baith o these babies were OK and Mrs L's bairns were aa at the school and they were fine. I wis wi the little eenies and her next door.

Fan it wis obvious that the bairn wisna gaan ti be lang, I wid get the husband to go fur the doctor. Sometimes he wis late. Often the baby wis there afore he arrived.

Fan I wis gaan tae deliver a baby, the thing wis maist o the hooses hid nae watter. We hid an ootside well. We used tae hae a fire on an twa big kettles an sometimes a pot hingin on the swye as weel. Ye aye needed a lot o het watter. An we'd oor tools an nappies, aathing ready fur the baby. I didna often dae the cuttin o the cord. I waited fur the doctor. I hiv deen't in an emergency, but that first een I wouldna ha dared cut it.

Anither woman wi a young faimly doon aside Stonehaven didna hae labour pains. She wis needin a cup o tea an her man wis in the hoose an aa. He wis gan tae ging through fur it an she says, 'Oh I'll get it masel'. Ye ken, independent. She stretched up tae get the tea an the baby arrived. Jist lik at. Nae warnin at aa. It knocked its heidie. We got the doctor an aathin. I got an afa shock. She didna hae a pain ye see. The doctor said I'd tae gie the baby wan drop o whisky in a teaspoonfae o its Mam's milk. I aye gaed it jist wan drop o whisky. I wis wi her aboot three wiks as she jist wisna afa weel. I na ken if it wis the quick delivery. The baby wis daein fine, thrivin. I wisna a wik hame fan I got word the baby hid deet. I wint doon a wee whilie efter tae see fit hid happened til the baby. She said, 'Well I've aye been giein it its wan drop o whisky'. She didna realise she'd been giein it a taespoonfu o whisky. She gave it the raw whisky an chokit the baby. She didna ken hersel how she did it. I'd aye been gi'in it an should ha been tellin her but ye'd think they wid ken. I regretted that I didna keep sayin mind jist one drop. Ye think Mams 'll ken. It wis afa sad. That wis afore the war.

I had my son Gordon so any time I hid tae ging oot I took him intae ma mither. Bill ma husband wis five and a half year a prisoner-of-war. I wis kept real busy wi the bairns. The pey wis jist naethin then. Fan I stairted it wis five shillings a wik. Then it gaed up. I think it wis aboot ten shillins fur a lot o the babies. Some o the folk couldna afford at. Ye aye hid yer food an yer bed wi them. But the money didna seem tae be important. As lang as I could dae fit I wis needed tae dae.

Anither ane up at Auchnagatt wis a nurse afore she wis married, an afa nice body. She says, 'Can ye jist come a wik or so afore if ye can?' I couldna get aff until just a few days afore the baby wis born. It wis quite a straightforward kin a birth. I delivered the baby. The doctor wis ere – he cam in aboot jist as the baby wis born. He wis a lovely baby.

Efter the baby wis aboot a wik aul, she took a haemor-rhage. She'd nivver been doon the stairs and she stairted ti come doon an she haemorrhaged. There wis twa young lads workin at the place an I shouted tae her hubby, 'Could ye get the doctor or come an gie me a help wi her first'. She wis lyin on the stair wi her feet doon. He pit in the twa loons – aboot fifteen they were – tae help an they cairried her up the stairs. I got them tae pit the bed up on books an I pit het watter bottles roon her. She wis oot fur the coont. I wis really worried aboot her. She nivver really recovered. She died aboot a year efter, she'd gotten her feet again but she kept takin these haemor-rhages.

Afore at, ae mornin aboot five, I wis up wi her or the baby, and we wis spikkin oboot the baby an she said, 'Do you think my baby's een are aa richt?' An I'm sayin, 'Well, I dinna ken. They are a bittie pale lookin'. I didna ken fit tae think. The doctor hid been called oot tae somebody an he saw the lichts on an I heard a rap at the door. 'Fa is at?' He came up tae see if onything wis wrang. She said til him, 'We're jist lookin at the baby's een. Div ye think they're aa richt?' So he looked an he says, 'Well, I have my doubts. He could be blind'. But he wisna sure. But he wis absolutely blin. The baby wis jist aboot a wik aul at this point. Now he's one o the heid anes at, it used to be caa'ed the Blind Asylum in Aiberdeen. I bedd wi her for a wee while.

At wis an afa sad time. The next woman I wis gaan tae be wi, her baby wis due in three wiks. This woman – her mother took her hame wi her. She couldna be left. I couldna bide langer because I had promised this ither ane. That wis the plan at the time. The next een wis so happy. She says, 'I've proved them aa wrang. I've aye been telt I couldna hae a family and here's me three wiks fae haein the baby'. An she took a brain haemorrhage and died at wik. I wisna there as I wis still wi this baby that wis blin. She nivver hid her baby. She would maybe ha been aboot twenty-eight. We were jist devastated. She wis sittin at her breakfast ae mornin. That wis afore the war. It put me aff a bittie because I thocht it could happen and me there, but it didna. There wis sad things bit a lot a happy things tae.

There wis ane ower at Slains again. It wis jist quite an ordinary birth. She'd a young faimly and she only died this year. I delivered her as well. I jist learned as I gid alang. Fan the doctor came he did the needfu but they didna get a lot o attention then. Nae pain relief.

After the baby was born I looked after the mam. I washed her and saw that she wis comfortable. The bairn too – I bathed the bairns. Maist o them breastfed. I can only min wan that didnae. I jist liked fit I wis daein There wis anither ane at Aden. It's a great place Aden. The hooses are aa made intil picture hooses an aathin noo wi big shops. She says, 'Will ye manage tae come tae me? Somebiddy telt me aboot ye'. I said, 'Oh aye, that'll be OK if I'm free'. Sometimes I wisna. Well I couldna tak twa on at ae time except that ither time an I didna ken I wis takken twa on at eence. So I wis wi her and it wis fine but again she seemed to hae jist an afa easy time. The baby arrived wi jist nae problems at aa.

Aa the doctors didnae hae cars. A lot o them hid bikes or especially in the sna they hid horses. Dr Dixon used tae come roon on his skis at aa oors o the night in the storms. Oor auld doctor got a motor-bike an eence he got on't he didna ken foo tae stop it. The first time he gaed awa wi't he couldna mind fit tae dae. He said, 'I couldna think fit hanle tae touch. I wis gaan roon ere an I wis supposed tae be awa tae someplace an I couldna stop it and I jist came by an jist ran roon an gid up an by until the petrol stoppit'.

I used a bike usually. I biked for miles and miles. I wish I could dee it noo. In the hooses I jist wis lik a hoosekeeper. Did aathin. Funny enough that hoose far the baby wis blin there wis a maid there but she took the measles an she'd tae go awa so I wis jist left tae carry on. There wis that two lads comin in fur their meals as weel.

Some o the mothers winted tae lie in bed an some o them didna. But they were aye a few days in their bed. Sometimes aboot a wik. If they hid ither little anes they wanted tae get up. It aa dependit on the mother. Once they got up they were OK.

Another woman had fourteen o a faimly. I min aboot her afa weel because it wis the time that Bill wis a prisoner an there wis a prisoner o war meetin. Her baby wisna due an I gid doon tae see her tae see aboot gaan tae be wi her. I said, 'There's a prisoner o war meetin on fitivver day it wis. But, I winna ging if ye're, ye ken'. She says, 'Oh no, fan I stairt, I tak ma time. Even if I'm stairtin ye wid hae time tae ging'. I gid doon tae see her in the mornin an I says, 'Will I ging or will I bide?' If ye gid tae the prisoner o war meetins ye sometimes heard somethin aboot yer man. An she says, 'Na, na, I'll be OK'.

So I gid tae the meetin. I wisna so lang awa really, jist aboot an oor, nae lang on the bus. Comin hame, there wis a lassie at the front o the bus an she wis sittin greetin. I didna ken her at aa. Fan I cam aff the bus, this lassie cam aff as weel an her dad wis ere meetin her. This wis this woman's husband. I didna ken him or the daughter. She had had the baby, nae warnin at aa, an she'd made fur her bed an she haemorrhaged an the baby wis OK but she wis away. She deet. Nae kennin aa this, I gid doon at nicht tae see fit like she wis. I couldna believe it an the baby wis lyin ere an she wis away. Three little eenies at hame and three at the school. I just took ower the hoose-keepin because I wis gaan there onywey but it wis an afa sad hoosehold. I wis ere a good whilie lookin efter them and then this lassie, her at wis at the bus greetin, she took ower fan I left, fan Bill cam hame. It wis terrible.

The bairn wis OK. There wis naebiddy ere fan she hid the bairn. An I wis spikkin til her in the mornin and she jist said, 'Oh I've plenty time. Go intil yer meetin'. Her husband found her. There wis an afa lot o blood by the fireside and the bed. I dinna ken fa gid in and picked the baby up. The aulest girl wis mairriet an she hersel wis expectin a baby at the time. And there wis a that eens nae grown up yet – three nae at the school. Peggy took ower an she wis good. I wis ere for the funeral an at an she kept singin, 'I'll walk alone'. Her hert wis jist full. She couldna spik I dinna think. It wis an afa bonny baby. Naebiddy ivver found oot if she kent that the baby wis alive.

There wis somebody else that wis needin me jist immediately efter at an I couldna. I jist couldna think aboot it. I'd a raither gin awa an yet I wouldna ha bin ere onywey because there wis nae phones. An if her man hid been oot.

Ye got used tae goin into the hooses. Ye could mak yersel at hame and jist tak ower. I think my longin tae be a nurse made me lik fit I wis at at time.Ye jist hid til get on wi't. Eence I got stairted wi at first baby I jist seemed tae wint tae dae it. I did work in atween times but I didna really hae a steady job because I aye had somebody waitin on me.

I did hae some wi the cord roon the neck but never as bad as that first een. It wis afa, the tightness o the cord ye ken tae get ma finger in, it wis jist . I wis feart I wid hurt the baby pushin her back. I kent she seemed tae be OK efter she yelled but I wondered if I hid daen ony ill tae her. But the doctor said no. He said probably ye could ha lost the baby and maybe her an aa. He wis afa nice aboot it. And then he recommended me.

8

FROM THE OUTER HEBRIDES

Canadian Boat Song
(The Lone Sheiling)

From the lone shieling of the misty island
Mountains divide us and the waste of seas –
Yet still the blood is strong, the heart is Highland,
And we in dreams behold the Hebrides!
Fair these broad meads, these hoary woods are grand;
But we are exiles from our fathers' land.

John Galt 1779–1839

*This midwife, who has asked not to be named, was born in
the Outer Hebrides in 1910 and lives there in retirement. She
did general nurse training in Edinburgh Royal Infirmary in
the early 1930s, then Queen's Nurse Training and was
seconded in 1939 by the Queen's Institute of District Nursing
to do midwifery training in the Montrose Maternity Hospital
in Govan. She completed district midwifery training in Edinburgh and practised as a Queen's Nurse in Central Scotland.
In 1945 she trained as a health visitor and worked in health
visiting before going to Glasgow to the Central Training
Institute for Queen's Nurses.*

*The Outer Hebrides have always been home to this mid-
wife and she chose'The Canadian Boat Song' to start this
chapter. She returned regularly to see her family and twice to
practise: once in 1944 to do 'double duties' as midwife and
district nurse and again for ten years in the fifties and sixties
to do 'triple duties' – midwife, district nurse and health
visitor. This chapter covers some of her experiences of working in the Outer Hebrides.*

On district, one was on call all the time. We didn't even have days off – just half days. The doctor would say,'Och, I think you're needing a day off'. So it was hard but I was happy when I got used to it. I had a car. Learn to drive was one of the first things I did when I started on district in 1940.

I did the antenatal care all the time and sometimes on the first visit the mother would say, 'There's another one on the way but don't tell the doctor yet'. I would say, 'But I must tell the doctor'. The doctor went after you notified him. They didn't book early. After that we visited fortnightly, and weekly for the last month. We were on call when they came to term. They phoned or sent a message and we went out to assess the situation. We asked them to contact us if they weren't sure, early in the day, because you had your work to plan. We told them where we were going to be. Sometimes we just had to stay where we were as there were lots of places without roads. You had to leave your car and walk the rest of the way.

One patient, para ten, lived in a small, scrupulously clean house off the road, up on the hill. I arrived about mid-day and she was walking about. I'd asked about previous labours and she said, 'Slow, but at the end one, two, three pains and there's the baby'. When I got the doctor in the afternoon he didn't examine her. He sat on a couch at the window and said, 'Oh well, here you are. You look fine to me'. She was making pancakes and scones and offered him a cup of tea. He had a talk with me and then asked the husband when the morning high tide was expected. 'Well', he said, 'it's now three o'clock. The tide will be at half past two to three in the morning.' So the doctor said, 'The good midwives long ago went by that. When they were called they looked at the tide. The baby will be born at three in the morning. I'm away then. You're in good hands'.

I did some visits down a back road. The evening came and the husband and her daughter went to bed. I said, 'You go to bed and have a rest'. She said, 'You could come in beside me'. I answered, 'I'd be stroked off the midwives Roll'. 'You know', she said, 'This is how I've been all the time. I'll tell you when it's coming.'

From the Outer Hebrides

At about a quarter to three in the morning, there was, 'Ah-h, ah-h', and then she said, 'Nurse, it is coming'. And she started – and the baby was born at about three a.m. Number ten. And it was the tide!

I waited for an hour after baby was bathed and came home. Later, I was doing an afternoon visit. I was by the fire wrapping up the baby. She said to me, 'Wasn't the doctor good? How he knew when the baby would come'. I nearly dropped the baby. 'Well', I said, 'I like that. The doctor's getting the praise, and here's me, I've more grey hairs today than I had when I came yesterday forenoon. He left me with all the worry.' She was so apologetic. 'Oh,' she said, I don't mean that. Oh love.' Each time I did my child welfare visit she would say, 'Oh have you forgiven me?' 'There's nothing to forgive,' I would say. Wasn't the doctor good! But she didn't mean it that way. Happy memories.

A young girl came from the mainland to have her baby at her granny's. There was the granny, the grandfather, her aunt, the aunt's husband and a little girl, in a thatched house but very orderly and clean. The first time I saw her, I thought, 'She's got a breech' and notified the doctor. We both went and he said, 'Oh no, that's not a breech. There's the head down there'. Of course I was asking myself, is the doctor right or am I?

I antenataled her twice over a fortnight and I was still convinced it was a breech. There were no phones and somebody came to my door to call me at about two in the morning. I had to walk quite a distance over a hilly area, carefully using the torch. I found her very advanced in labour. There was meconium staining and her uncle was dispatched for the doctor about eight to ten miles away. He had to go quite a bit to the next house and waken the neighbour who had a car. The baby was born and I had tidied up before the doctor arrived. The mother was very co-operative and I remembered all my breech teaching and techniques. It was a bed in the wall with a flock mattress. The girl's aunt who was there was very sensible and intelligent. I got everything I needed considering that they had no mod cons, and only water from the well.

However, the baby was very white and limp and I was very anxious. The aunt said, 'Don't worry, the mother is alive and that's the main thing'. I asked, 'Have you any whisky?' Perhaps they thought *I* was needing it. I put a little on cotton wool and put it up to the nostrils and the baby gasped and I believe it helped although other people perhaps don't think so. So the baby survived.

I went away to do my health visitor training and in the lectures we got some midwifery. One day we were having breech. That baby was still at the back of my mind. I listened intently to 'the breech' and the danger of the after-coming head. Fortunately this baby was small, just seven pounds. We spoke about resuscitation and the lecturer said, 'Just resuscitate them even although you may think they're not with you. Keep them warm'.

I still worried about that baby and whether she had been brain-damaged. One time, about five years later, I saw the granny and asked how things were. She told me my little one was at school and doing well. However, I was determined I would see for myself. I was going south and I knew the father worked on the railway. I found the house and the mother came to the door but she didn't remember me. I said, 'Do you remember seeing me on on the 16th of December 1944?' She took my hands in hers and she had my name. I told her I wanted to see the wee girl I had delivered and when she came in – I did an assessment! She was absolutely fine and I believed them that time. It eased my mind.

I delivered quite a number of babies at home. In 1944-45 in isolated areas there weren't many homes with mod cons. After the war, things changed very quickly because there were grants for home improvements. In 1944-45 there were no phones but in the fifties the phones had come and there was a car! Numbers of deliveries varied. There could be two in a week and several in a month. It depended on the size of the area. During the war there were quite a lot away in the Services. It was an ageing population even then and very scattered.

One mother who had several children went to hospital

with placenta praevia. The husband came for me thinking she was in labour and it was then I became very suspicious. It was something about the palpation, possibly a high head. I wrote a note and sent for the doctor. He didn't come but ordered an ambulance. I went with her by ambulance to hospital and eventually a live baby was born. When there was only one doctor and one nurse in the area you had to have confidence in each other.

Most of my deliveries were normal. Later, doctors were more inclined to send mothers into hospital although they preferred being at home. I felt disappointed because mid-wifery was very enjoyable on the district. It was lovely to have a new baby and wonderful with the baby born at home and the rest of the family there. The fathers weren't at the delivery then.

There were quite a number of big families. The population has gone down since then. One doctor was quite happy about babies being born at home unless there was some reason. Perhaps nobody available to help. They didn't have home helps then. When a new doctor came he said after the fourth they would go to the hospital. Mothers were then sent in for the first delivery. He was young and decided it was safer for the mother to be in hospital.

My maternity case was always in the car and we had our pack which we made up containing gown, masks, bonnet, cotton wool and swabs. The pack was untouched until it was opened in the house for the confinement. It was amazing. There were always children around and we wrapped the pack up in brown paper and put it on top of a cupboard. Nothing was ever touched.

Mothers were in bed for ten days – I don't know if they stayed in bed when we were gone but they were kept in bed and we did everything. We went in and took the temperature, measured the fundus and all the rest and bathed them for three days. Then later on as conditions improved in the houses they could get up for a bath.

I also bathed the baby for ten days but if it was a first baby I showed the mother how to manage, to give her confidence.

There was always a granny or someone volunteering to look after the baby but I didn't like that. I preferred to do it myself as I wanted to watch the cord and continue the routine until the tenth day and perhaps go back afterwards if there were any feeding problems. They always seemed to do well.

In the olden times the mother really stayed in bed – she didn't come out of bed at all in the first ten days, we are told! The friends went before she got up, to see the mother and the baby and there is an old Gaelic word for it: 'Bàngaid', which is like banquet. It is pronounced 'banget' with a grave accent on the first A. They went at night to these bàngaids. It was war time with the blackout and you had to carry a torch upside down. No roads down to some places. They got a glass of wine. One time, around 1942-44 there was a confinement. The husband said to me, 'You know how we have a bangaid? It's difficult to get wine'. I think it might have been port. He said, 'You know this is the custom. Will you give me a line? Write a line for me to take so that I can get some wine?' I said, 'A line for you to get wine? I'd be shipped off on the boat next week without any work'. 'Oh but,' he said, 'they used to ' I said, 'They who? Who was that?' He didn't say another thing but he was huffy for a wee while but got over it.

I wasn't invited to the bàngaids which weren't big gatherings. It was just a small community and it was mostly the older married ladies who went. They came with a wee present and got tea and wine. It was an old, old custom, and usually at night.

You know those women they called the howdies. I didn't work with any howdies but in 1942-44 I did meet one where the ladies had the bàngaids. Two men came for me early one morning. In that district, they had to walk across a moor with only a path, to a village by the shore, get a motor boat and cross over to where the doctor and the nurse were. So they had all that way to come and then return with me. By the time I arrived, the baby was born and a howdie was there. I still remember that handsome lady – she was eighty – and she was standing there and I said, 'Oh hello. Well, I'm glad you were here'. The mother was quite happy lying with the baby, and the first thing I thought, 'the cord'. She had covered the baby and when I looked the umbilical cord was intact. That was the trouble previously. They cut the cord. They would just say, 'Give me a pair of scissors'. But she had left it. She just said, 'I left everything for you nurse'. She had covered the baby and the baby was fine between the mother's legs. The mother was very happy. 'Oh,' she said to me, 'The baby's here!'

I remember that incident because I heard stories of howdies. The area I was in in Central Scotland as a health visitor had one and although I never met her, I heard she was very loath to give up. She was kind and *she* wanted to deliver the babies. I think some of the certified midwives had battles with her. She would say, 'Oh you've time enough to send for the midwife'. Then she would be able to deliver the baby.

On one of the islands there was a patient, who had booked with my relief, waiting for me to visit her. When I visited, she said she was due in about ten weeks but she didn't appear as much as that. When I examined her there was no baby. I told her I would have a talk with the doctor. 'Is there anything wrong?' she asked. I said, 'Are you sure of your dates because you should be much bigger than you are?' 'Oh yes,' she said, 'I'm sure of my dates. That's happening every month.' When I told the doctor he asked what I thought. 'Well,' I said, 'There's no baby there.' He said we would see her one day soon.

A while after that the doctor said, 'We'll have to go and see that patient. Her husband was here, and he said his wife was complaining that she couldn't bend to close her shoe laces now'. He was going to take us both by boat but the day we were to go, I was held up and I was away on holiday the following week and couldn't do anything about it. The doctor said, 'I'll see her,' and added, 'I'll just ask her husband to take her over to the surgery'. I went away on holiday. She went to a mainland hospital and that was that.

In due course I got a letter from her booking for confinement. She was very apologetic about the previous incident. I visited her and there was a baby this time. She had a few children after that. It's very rare, isn't it? She was desperate to have a baby. Pseudocyesis is really strange. Truly, we are fearfully and wonderfully made.

In one place, still wartime, it was a first baby. There was no phone but I was able to notify the doctor and he came in the late evening. Time dragged on and eventually he said, 'I don't want to do it but if she goes on like this I think we'll have to have a forceps delivery'. After that the patient was a bit quieter. I can't criticise because I haven't been in labour but Doctor was saying she was very impatient. She was in bed and continually calling me. The doctor told her, in a kind way, that it was only her first baby and she would have to learn to have more patience. Then in the early hours we heard a noisy engine outside, opened the upstairs window and someone said, 'Is the doctor there? The District Nurse wants him for a confinement at the other end of the island'. Doctor said to me, 'I'll have to go, see what you can do with her'. So, after that the granny (her mother- in-law), who had had seven babies, a lovely lady, she came up and said to me, 'You haven't even had tea. Come down and have something'. The table was laid with scones, oatcakes, crowdie. She went over and said to the mother, 'We all know the first baby doesn't come easily. You'll have to have patience. It's not going to hurry. We'll go down. You come and go on your knees by the bed'. Well, the baby was born at half-past- nine in the morning, a spontaneous delivery. So there you are – nothing new under the sun.

Another time, the phone rang. It was a freezing cold, late afternoon. Someone in the post office in another village phoned and said, 'There's a message here for you'. (The midwife for that area was away.) 'The mother says her daughter is having pain in her back.' She added quietly, 'Bring your maternity bag'. I said, 'I have that in the car all the time'.

It was a first baby. I notified the doctor and he arrived. It was a very hard frost. We were there late afternoon and evening. The doctor was very patient but he couldn't move because of the frost and snow and we had to stay there all night. When it came to about seven in the morning, he said, 'I must try and get to the surgery'. They managed to get him on to the road and he went away. After that, the patient said, 'Could I have a cigarette? I'm just dying for a cigarette'. I said, 'I have never had that request before from someone in labour'. I eventually gave in and said she could have one. She lit up and looked so relaxed. I think we nearly fell asleep! There were just the two of us and we were quiet. Shortly after that contractions came. She delivered quickly. I left a message for the doctor that the baby was born and mother and baby satisfactory. Doctor asked, 'How did you manage that?' So I told him.

I felt really isolated as a district nurse in remote areas especially during the war. You were at it all day and didn't get to know people. People were very kind. You had to be available twenty-four hours a day. Before there were phones you left a message on a slate inside the window giving your location. Then people could see it and know where you were to be found.

The midwife attended postnatally for ten days, then fourteen days and again back to ten when the CMB Rule changed again. But the midwife could go in for longer, up to twenty eight days if necessary. That was the CMB Rule.

I don't remember any postnatal infections. They were in their own homes and we were trained to have very high standards of cleanliness and watch for cross-infection. One tutor was impressing on us the importance of cleanliness. She said, 'I discovered when you were called to a mother, everything would be in order but the feet were always dirty'. So she said, 'The first thing you did was to wash the feet'. She told us a story about a little boy who was going to bed when first the district nurse came and then his granny came. He got a little sister and was all excited. When he went to school next morning his teacher said, 'Oh, Johnny, aren't you fortunate getting a little sister?' He answered, 'Well, you see, please Miss, it's very easy. You just wash your feet and send for your Granny'.

Most mothers breastfed but as time went on artificial feeding became popular. There were mothers who said, 'I can't breastfeed'. Some who were keen and anxious to do it couldn't cope. Some mothers said, 'I wouldn't have time to sit down and breastfeed'. I think that was often the reason. But they get a rest when they are breastfeeding. Some mothers didn't want to do it.

To care for the cord we had a binder and a dusting of Johnson's baby powder. In the early days we pinned the binder, later we sewed it on and latterly we had adhesive tape to secure it.

Then the mothers – they had their binders too. They supplied their own – cotton or calico. If one didn't breastfeed, she got a binder firmly round her breast. The tutor told us that the best thing to use as a binder was a bolster-case and safety-pins to secure it. Quite a process.

Being in the triple role was ideal. You knew the mother. You were usually the first one to know if there was a baby coming and then you knew that baby, followed it up to five years and then at school. I had many years of the triple role and the continuity was marvellous. It was very rewarding and you felt you were part of the household. I lived in the nurse's house and drove the nurse's car. In the Outer Hebrides it was an A30, then a Ford and finally a little blue Mini – new!

At the time one didn't realise it but now as I reminisce, I think, 'Well it was a privilege'. In our lectures on the ethics of district nursing and midwifery we were told, however long you have been in a place, never just walk into a house. Always knock, then open, and ask, 'May I come in?' The privilege of being committed to serving and caring for people who needed and trusted you, makes me feel now that it was such an honour.

During the war I had a patient with a big family. Her son was away in the war in the army or navy – he was quite young – and just a few weeks before the baby was due, the son was killed. I remember the mother. She was very saddened and heartbroken. After the baby was born, a lovely little boy, she said, 'Well, it's wonderful. I was almost on the verge of losing my faith. This child has given me my faith back and the will to live'. So, you were sharing their sorrows and their joys.

9

ANNE CHAPMAN

Anne Chapman was born in 1917 and trained as a midwife in Glasgow Royal Maternity Hospital, known to many as Rotten Row. Much of her midwifery practice was done amongst travelling folk in and around Glasgow. In this chapter, she tells of some of these experiences. Anne lives in Auchtermuchty, Fife and writes poetry in Scots.

I felt very honoured to be able to go to Rotten Row. I know lots of girls who were turned down because too many applied. The matron and the tutor interviewed me and I took to the tutor straight away. This was me as a qualified nurse going into midwifery in 1939 or 1940 at the start of the war. Glasgow wasn't too involved in the war then. Later on all the stushie came and the blackouts. I stayed an extra year as a midwife because I wanted the experience. I was really pleased to make my life's work in midwifery and to be able to teach girls who came from other countries. Coloured girls from all over the world. Most of them came from Africa because there were no hospitals there to train them. I felt proud when they passed their finals to think they were able to do this job and they were going to do it in their own country.

They must have seen Glasgow as a big change from their homeland. Some of them had been in hospitals down south doing general nursing. They couldn't follow what people were saying. If the patient said something, they would say, 'What's she saying?' and I had to tell them. We were really in among the poorest of the poor. People that had any money at all used to pay to go to nursing homes.

We went to Glasgow Green where all the gypsy tents were and to the dunnies. That's the Scottish word for the dungeon.

These people were travellers and they would move around in caravans. Most of them had quite big families and needed a place to stay in the winter. They came back to Glasgow and their caravans would probably be put on Glasgow Green or wherever, and they got the dunny underneath the tenements. You went in the tenement building and instead of going up you went down. The dunnies were mostly empty in the summertime. Every tenement had them. The dunny was the whole stretch of the tenement underneath with no division, just long areas under the tenements with trodden earth floors. The people would move in. Some of them had sacking and they could put up sacks or whatever they had to curtain it off. It made it a wee bit more private. There would be a family on each side.

At least twice I was down the dunny delivering. Some of them were used as stores. One time, I said, 'What am I smelling?' and the mother told me a fruiterer stored his potatoes there. Somewhere else, a garage kept spare parts in the dunny. When you went to deliver them you just used any thing you could get. Sometimes the babies were delivered on to a heap of rags. If they had a camp bed they were considered posh. My mother wouldn't believe me when I was telling her that.

We were often called out at night and then we usually had a medical student with us. They might be at lectures during the day at university and they weren't there when the calls came in and we had to be ready to jump and run. But through the night they were always there. There were a lot of different students from England, Italy, Africa and Canada. One, an American, thought the way the people had to live was awful. He was fascinated when I told him about their caravans and they went travelling in the summer away over Scotland, England and Ireland and came back in the winter. A caravan wouldn't have been warm enough in the winter to have a baby in. I remember one of the nights going down into the dunny and I was wondering how we were going to see and there were bottles sitting around with candles in. I think they had one of these old black stoves for heating in the dunnies. I remember boiling water on it but they only used it when they needed it.

We were often in the caravans on Glasgow Green. They were in a different street and were very clean. I used to wonder how they kept them so clean but I think the particular caravan you delivered the mother in was just kept special.

Every mother breastfed. I didn't come across many people, no matter where they delivered in Glasgow, that didn't breastfeed. It was the cheapest way to do it. There weren't the hand-outs in these days. It was long after that that dried milk came on to the market. Sometimes cows' milk would be used, watered down and with sugar in it but I never encouraged that. If the mother said, 'I'm going to try', I gave her all the encouragement. The mothers didn't have jobs to run to like the young ones nowadays. They want to get back to their job and Granny will take the baby. Then it needs to be fed away from the mum and this is the result. I was very sad about it because I felt breastfeeding was the best.

We had to walk everywhere. However, an awful lot of places in Glasgow got their refuse emptied during the night. We used to stand up on the back of the refuse-cart and get a lift. They didn't do it in every area. They had a long platform on the back of the cart and through the day the men would stand on that but at night there was only the driver and one man and he could get into the cab. If the driver saw us he would stop and yell, 'Where are ye goin?' and he would take us. One time we were walking to Springburn and that was a long road away. 'We're going to Springburn.' 'Jump on'. And there we were clutching on the back – the student and I. Rattling away and then he would shout, 'What street are ye goin to?' These men were great.

Only a few of the midwives had bikes but as well as walking we could use the trams. The hospital issued tokens for tramcars which were doled out at the beginning of the month. At night there was nothing for it but to walk. One time, very early in the morning we were walking back from Springburn to the hospital when the first tram came along. We flagged it down and the driver let us on. But he obviously didn't want to stop again because he said, 'Jump in and spread yersels oot and look like a lot o folk!'

All this time, and I was out many a night, I never came across anybody that frightened me. If I maybe heard the footsteps passing I never ever thought anything about saying 'Good evening' or whatever. There are no slums in the middle of Glasgow now. They've built all these houses outside the city and done away with them.

I used to go to lots of gypsies' tents and caravans out in the rural areas. They always had dogs. Alsatians that I'm sure would have swallowed you alive if you let them. Once I went to a quarry. I had a lot of bother finding this place but I'll never forget it. There was just one entrance into it and they had tents all round. There was a dog's kennel at one side of the entrance and a dog's kennel at the other and two of the most ferocious Alsatians I have ever seen in my life. When anybody came near, they came out barking and growling and baring their teeth. They were tied so they couldn't meet each other but you could never have passed through this small space between them. I was terrified. The first time I went I was on my bicycle. I stood and called and shouted. Somebody was supposed to be in labour but nobody came. Then I saw children and they came. I said, 'Find one of the ladies'. One of them said, 'Is it ma granny ye're wantin?' and I said, 'Well your granny'll do fine'. The granny appeared and one word fae her and these dogs went slinking into their kennels. I couldn't believe it. Then she said, 'Noo nurse come on, bring yer bike. Somebody might lift it leavin it there'.

This was me on my own in this old quarry and the tents all round a big fire in the middle where they did their cooking. These really ugly dogs were still howling and barking because I was the stranger and they would smell me but one word from her and they were away and they never came back out until I was away pedalling on my bike. It's amazing how they're trained.

When it was all over and the baby was born and everything was grand the Granny said, 'Ye'll need tae get a cup o tea'. It was out of a tin can. You never said no because you wouldn't want anyone to think you were feeling a bit uppity. They were always so grateful and wanted to give you tea or whatever they had. There was always the camp fire going outside the caravans and tents with the kettle or tinnie on the boil. One time I had delivered the baby, the water had been boiled for the baby's first bath and I was ready to get on my bike and get back to the hospital, not forgetting the placenta. The mother had been given a syrup tin of tea and the grandfather who was really proud of the bairn turned and said, 'A drink o tea. Ye'll tak it'. I couldn't refuse. 'Hae a seat.' I sat down on the ground and was handed a tinnie of tea with a handle. But the tinnie had been on the fire and my mouth was badly burnt. I never said a word. By the next day I had to report to Sister. I couldn't go out because of my sore mouth. An old doctor looked me up and down very severely and said: 'What have you been doing to your mouth?' I said the first thing that came into my head, 'One of the doctors kissed me'. What a long time I took to live that one down.

I delivered a baby in a tent on the floor. They gave me a clean blue sheet for the delivery. They always had clothes for the baby, not new but they were always washed, maybe not ironed but always clean, and a shawl or a blanket or whatever, to wrap round the baby afterwards.

Another time, I was going to a caravan and this one big dog was tied up on a long stretch of rope at the side of the caravan. I was just paying a visit, the mother hadn't had her baby but the doctor had asked somebody to call as she was bloated with water, and he wanted one of us to go and have a talk to her and tiptoe round the subject of going to hospital. You couldn't just go in and say, 'You're going to hospital'.

This big dog came out barking and yowling. I was frightened and just stood stock still. This man came out. 'Come on, nurse, come on.' I still stood. and he said, 'It micht bite ye but it'll no hurt ye'. I said, 'Well I would rather it was inside'. So he grabbed the chain and held on till I got past. 'It micht bite ye but it'll no hurt ye'. When I went back I told one of the others about that and said, 'Don't be frightened to go in there because the dog might bite ye but it'll no hurt ye'. They were in hysterics.

Another time, I was attending a lady called Mrs MacDonald. She was in a caravan when she had her baby, I had delivered her and this was postnatally. She had a wee bit of trouble with breast feeding. I told the sister on the district who went and saw her and then said to me, 'I think that woman will have to stop breastfeeding. Tell her to get Nestlé's milk'. That was another great thing and they watered it down. I don't think breastfeeding was helping the baby in this case. It was fractious and crying a lot and right enough once it went on to the bottle there was no more trouble. The mother got a handful of pills to take three times a day. Sister said, 'If you feel she's going to need more, let us know'. So I said to her quite the thing, 'By the way, Mrs. MacDonald, is yer peels gaan tae see ye oot?' She said to me very indignantly, 'Nurse, my name's MacDonald but I dinna hae the Gaelic'. I never let on it wisna Gaelic. When I went home I told Sister who came from the Western Islands – Sister Stewart. She thought that was hilarious. She said it's good to find a wee bit of humour in places like that.

One night a medical student and I went to do a delivery in a tenement building. They all had gas mantles for lighting usually fixed to the mantlepiece. It was never very high and you had to watch you didn't knock your head on it. The student had been out at a dance the night before and he was tired. He said to me, 'I'm going to sit down on this chair and shut my eyes. Give me a shout when the head appears'.

I was encouraging the mother to get on with her delivery and all of a sudden the waters broke and I could see the head was crowning and I shouted tae him. He jumped up and put his head through the mantle and left us all in darkness. I never let him forget that and there's me delivering this baby in blackout. Then they had to run and look for candles.

Canada not only sent medical students. During the Second World War, there came what became known as 'Canada parcels'. These ware parcels of clothes for babies from the Canadian people as a gift to Scotland during the war years. People really appreciated that.

Usually as I left a newly delivered mother and her baby she would say, 'Good bye, nurse, see you next year'.

10

ALICE MAY BRODIE PORTER

Alice Porter trained as a midwife in Aberdeen in 1939–40. She didn't keep a record, but said she must have delivered between eight or nine hundred babies. Alice latterly lived in California and told these anecdotes for this oral history collection to her friend, Mary Gilhooley, in 1997. Alice died, at the age of eighty-seven, on 13 August, 2000.

During the Second World War I was instructed to go to George Street in Aberdeen. I couldn't find the place and the whole area looked deserted. I finally found a policeman who said, 'There's no-one living here. These houses have been condemned'. The windows had been blown out and the stairways were blown out and had no banisters. We heard a noise and went up a stair to find a young woman on a couch – no blankets or sheets. Over by an empty fireplace was an old woman smoking a clay pipe and spitting into a fireplace. I asked her if there was any water in the building. She said 'No' but made no move to help me. I couldn't leave the young woman so I asked the policeman to come back in a couple of hours. I had to pour a bottle of Dettol on my hands before I examined the woman. I sat in a chair with a rim but no seat until it was time to deliver the child.

Just before the child was born the sirens sounded and the blast blew out the sacking covering the windows and soot blew into the room from the roofs. Under these conditions I delivered the baby. The policeman arrived with an ambulance, I carried the new baby down the broken stairway to the waiting ambulance, and mother and child were transported to hospital.

These people were referred to as tinkers – I suppose nowadays they would be squatters or homeless.

I was sent to deliver a baby in Hutcheon Street in Aberdeen and to make three follow-up visits. On the fourth day I was to ask for the fee which was five shillings and take it back to the sister in charge. When I asked for the fee, the mother said, 'Pay it yourself'. I didn't know what to do so I went home to my mother who gave me the five shillings. When I took it to the Sister she said, 'You must have got that from your mother – that woman has had four deliveries and has never paid. Take the money back to your mother'.

Still in wartime Aberdeen:

I once attended a patient who was rather belligerent and who had a little girl. I thought there was something a little different about the child, but didn't know what. The Sister said it might be a good idea to visit at a different time of day and see if the father was home. I did this and discovered the father was a coloured gentleman.

The sequel to this story was that about eight years later I was showing a colleague the maternity facilities in Aberdeen and the old Maternity Pavilion which had become a barracks. We came upon some children playing and stopped to talk to them and ask their names. One little girl who was darker than her companions informed me her name was – Alice May Brodie Porter. Midwives had to make out a Notification of Birth Certificate for every child they delivered and sign it. The mother maybe didn't like me much but she gave her little daughter my full name.

I was sent to Marischal Street in Aberdeen to attend an expectant mother and I had with me a young student doctor who was to be my pupil during the delivery. When the husband opened the door, he said, 'You can come in Doctor. *She* can't come in here – she's too young'.

I knew there was a Police Station at the foot of Marischal Street by the docks, so I walked down there in the rain. With the blackout I could hear the water lapping at the dock-wall but couldn't see anything. I called out, 'I need a policeman' and a voice answered, 'I'm a policeman. What do you need?'

We made our way back to the house and the policeman

told the prospective father, 'This is the woman who's going to deliver your child'.

When the baby was delivered, it had a caul over its head and face. I immediately removed it while explaining to the student what it was. The mother got quite excited and said to give it to her husband. Her husband was a seafaring man and sailors of course consider a baby's caul very lucky. He was so happy he insisted I sit down and have a glass of whisky. I never did drink spirits but I didn't want to upset him so I poured the whisky into a convenient aspidistra next to my chair. On my follow-up visit mother and baby were doing well, but the mother couldn't understand why her nice plant had suddenly died.

11

ELLA BANKS AND LINDA STAMP

Ella was born in Dunfermline in 1915 and Linda, in Glasgow in 1916. They were pupil midwives in the early 1940s. They both began their midwifery training at Glasgow Royal Maternity Hospital. (Rotten Row). However, Ella moved to Motherwell and finished her training there. Now, they both live in very active retirement in Wick.

ELLA When I did my general nurse training in Dunfermline, West Fife, which was a very good hospital we were treated as professional people. We put our shoes at the door to be cleaned by the maid every night. In the morning she knocked on the door and said, 'It's six o'clock nurse', and put your clean shoes in. When I went to Rotten Row I put my shoes out at the door! The next morning I woke up with such a clatter as my shoes were thrown in. 'Where do you think you are? The so-and-so Ritz?' We lived below the ground at Rotten Row. We were in a basement and all you could see when you looked out of the kind of narrow window was other people's feet. That was the nurses' home.

LINDA We paid £50 for our training, got no salary and had to buy our uniforms. My father had nothing to do with my training. He gave me my books and my uniform when I started but not a penny after that. My mother helped – she gave me half-a-crown a week until I was earning. If I needed to buy anything I borrowed the money and she took interest for it, telling me I would learn to value money. I paid her back after I was earning.

ELLA The food was terrible. Just great tins with what was left over from yesterday put in day after day and it was ladled on to your plate. There was a row of stony-faced sisters behind this servery with the ladles. We were very hungry. One day Linda said, 'I'm still hungry' after pudding and somebody dared her to ask for more. And she went up and asked for more pudding. You could have heard a pin drop in this great dining-room. Everybody was thunderstruck and these sisters just looked at one another and one took her ladle and plonked another dollop on her plate. After that they asked if anyone wanted more.

LINDA One thing pleased us. To make a little on the side, the cook used to save the dripping and put it in a jar and we could buy it for a shilling. We brought the jar back to her. We put the dripping on our bread – it was lovely. That was important at that time with rationing.

ELLA One night we were very hungry. My sister sent me a parcel every month with things I would need, like toothpaste and sanitary towels and always currant bun. We always shared parcels and we were having tea and currant bun when the Home Sister who we called Snow White came along. She found us and she was most annoyed and you [Linda] said to her, 'That's Nurse Young's currant bun we're eating and not the hospital's, and that's my mother's tea and tea pot'. The sister said, 'But it's the hospital gas you're using'.

ELLA The first week there, we were all sent to the labour ward to see a posthumous birth which we would never probably see again. The woman had just died and the baby was being delivered. The doctor asked us to go. However, one of the senior midwives ordered us all back to the ward – we shouldn't be standing there gazing.

LINDA Everything had to be done so quickly, like yesterday. I used to get so mixed up. One time I was running to the slunge with a pail of things to be slunged in my hand. At the same time I'd been told to get a glass of milk for the sister. I had so many conflicting orders that when I looked down there was no pail in my hand. I'd put it down somewhere. You must remember we were young and it was our first experience and it was pretty grim, it really was grim. I got such a shock suddenly realising that I'd no pail in my hand and I had to run back and get the pail. I was the mucker-up. When you were on slunge duty that was it. I remember that night. I was so tired.

I can tell you a tragic thing. In Rotten Row we had a venereal disease ward. They kept mothers with VD separate from the others. I was a bit of a troublemaker at the time. They [the mothers] got a bowl of soup and when they were finished you took the bowl back to the ward sister who was serving. I put the soup bowl down in the sink. We were all new to the ward. There was no permanent staff to tell us how things were done except the sister. She lifted the bowl off the sink and she dumped in the tatties and mince and I said, 'Oh sister, I haven't washed the bowl'. She never answered me. She said, 'Take that in to . . .' I said, 'I didn't wash it'. She paid no attention. 'Go and give her her dinner'. So I did. This went on for two or three days and we were all talking about it. I said, 'This is filth'. They got their pudding in the same bowl and the bowl was never washed. Well, on the third or fourth day I refused to do it. We had words and I was ordered to Matron. I got a telling off and I said, 'Well, it's unfortunate but I'm sorry, I couldn't do it. I get ill'. Things like that and smells always affected me. Matron asked if I wanted to make a formal complaint. I said, 'If it's necessary, I will'. The form was made out and I was told to sign it. I lifted the pen on the desk, and she said, 'That's my pen'. You can imagine me lifting the best fountain pen. I never heard another thing but I was shifted very soon.

Also in the VD ward, there was a woman who was in labour whose knees were up to her chin, but close together. Her knees opened automatically when she was about to deliver her baby and it was the most fantastic birth I have ever seen. It all happened so suddenly. They hadn't time to get her to the little theatre off the VD ward. It just suddenly happened. Sister came running and told me to go and phone. I came back and there were these legs – they were opening like that and it was a beautiful birth.

ELLA When the bombers went over the mothers and babies were put under the beds to give them even a little protection.

LINDA The midwives didn't get any special protection. You were always given work to do. We were always given something. I was in the labour ward and admission. There were four of us in the labour ward and admission with Sister McQueen. We had a very favourite name for her. She was a very good sister but she could fairly lash out so we had always to be occupied. We were always given work to do.

On the District

ELLA We were very obvious with straw hats with navy velvet and white ties under the chin and a navy blue coat. In a bus queue, in that uniform, they always pushed you to the front whether you were going on a case or not.

LINDA We got tokens for the tramcars but the calls always seemed to be at night when there were no tramcars running and we had to walk. I used to get so tired coming back in the early hours of the morning. I remember one morning sitting on the pavement waiting for the first tramcar to get back to Rotten Row.

After we had worked six weeks on the district we took the medical students out. They were training – doing their midder. Even as student midwives we supervised them doing their deliveries. After we came back from a delivery we had to do our cases up. Then we sat there making ties for umbilical cords. I think the sister just wanted to keep us occupied. We were never allowed to sit idle. To make the umbilical cords we had very fine white thread just like string. It had to be a certain length and we taped so many together. The sister for district was pretty old and very fussy. She supervised us and inspected our bags before we went out. Everything we took was essential. We had our sterile things in little packs. They weren't really sterile packs but they were washed and clean and clean towels and the umbilical cords.

We were always on the watch for anything abnormal and if necessary we contacted the hospital for help. Mostly you were left on your own and when we weren't doing deliveries we did postnatal visits, swabbing up and checking on the mothers. These were not necessarily our own postnatal cases. We often didn't know who we were going to see. We didn't do antenatal visits.

When we took some of the medical students out some funny things happened. Do you remember the time the cat ran away with the placenta?

ELLA We had to have a sponge bag with drawstrings, and in this, we had to put the placenta and bring it back to the hospital to be checked to see that it was complete and healthy.

LINDA The time the cat took the placenta my friend who'd delivered the baby ran after the cat and she did get some of it back, but not very much. She blamed the student. There were these three medical students we'd to be with, and we nicknamed them Faith, Hope and Charity. She had Charity with her on that occasion and she was very cross with him because he made no attempt to help her to catch the cat. But then he was possibly busy bathing the baby which he had to be supervised to do too.

LINDA My father was never ever keen on my being in nursing at all. He made himself clear three years before when I started my general training. When I started midwifery we got fleas. It was easily done. You were walking in and climbing on these wall beds – and I got fleas and then my father got fleas and so I was banned from the house. My mother used to come up to meet me in Pettigrew's for afternoon tea so everybody there probably got fleas too.

ELLA We'd to deliver the babies in those box-beds right into the wall so you just had to get up on a chair and kneel in the bed. I've delivered a baby and its Daddy wouldn't rise out of the bed to let his wife be delivered.

LINDA That was not uncommon. I've put a baby in a wooden drawer because there was nowhere else. Glasgow was poverty-stricken then. And the bandy legs. Dr Wattie worked so hard at that time to eliminate rickets.

Another thing. I remember the district-room sister telling us what to do with Roman Catholic families. If we were worried about the baby we had to send for the priest in case the baby died. You got laldy if you didn't get the priest in time to give the baby the last rites.

ELLA We delivered babies in houses where there was real poverty with nothing ready for the baby. No cot, blankets or clothes. I've wrapped many a baby in a towel and left it with its mother. Although they were so poor they were so friendly and helpful to one another. A neighbour would go round other neighbours with babies and get clothes for the new baby. Yet they couldn't be more hospitable. I've drunk tea out of a jam jar with a dry biscuit. They had to give us something.

When you delivered the baby, there was usually a neighbour there to hold the baby while you did what you'd to do to the mother. Then you had to see to the baby. We used oil to take off the vernix and then we bathed the baby and wrapped it in whatever was available and put it back in the bed beside the mother. Not all houses were destitute but there was no affluence around where I worked. Our district took in Motherwell and Wishaw and Craigneuk where there was a lot of unemployment. Sometimes baby clothes were waiting if you were very lucky. The baby very often just had a wooden drawer as a cot. But they were happy, and friendly, they helped one another and gave us a great welcome going back for our postnatal visits. We were received like royalty.

Quite often you were called to deliver a baby of a mother you'd never seen before. We did no antenatal visits so knew nothing about her – no notes or anything. This was as a student midwife going into homes by yourself. You had to diagnose for yourself how the baby was lying and what stage of labour she was at. One time, the mother was well into labour and when I palpated her abdomen, I thought, 'I've got a breech in there', and I had to deliver it. I had no calamities.

When I went in the next day they were always pleased to see me. I'd bath the baby again usually in a washing-up basin – sometimes just the sink. They were bathed and powdered and wrapped in what you could get.

I never had to call for help but I've had to send a message to the labour ward to say I was going to be a long time – if the mother wasn't very far on or if it was a very long labour. We did this, not because they would be worried about you but they might think you were swinging the lead. They never came to see that you were OK. Sometimes you had to spend all night with her, with primigravidas particularly. Once out, you stayed and the hospital knew where you were and we took it for granted that that was what we had to do. We went on a wing and a prayer, I suppose, but we managed it and I never heard of anybody getting into any real difficulties.

Some of the fathers weren't very savoury. Box-beds were commonly used and one father in particular wouldn't get out of the bed to let his wife be delivered in peace. He just wasn't a bit interested in his wife producing another member of the family. Some had to be put out as they were so excited but fathers weren't allowed to be at the birth in those days . . .

One mother was in one of those very high box-beds and I had to stand on a chair to get anywhere near her. We were getting on and were at the final stages with the head showing when the door opened and in rushed two little children pulling at my legs, 'What are ye daein tae my Mam?' I had to say, 'Just go away. Your Mum's all right'. The poor woman was saying, 'Go outside just now. I'm all right'.

There was no analgesic or gas and air. Mothers having a normal labour at home seemed to cope better with pain. I think they thought this is the natural thing to do. This is what we as women are here for and they just got on with it. Any roaring and shouting I've heard have been in a labour ward in hospital. On the district I've had them saying they were exhausted and they'd had all they could take but there were no loud shouts. Hospitals frighten people.

The hospital didn't supply bicycles but two or three of the student midwives had bikes and appeared willing to share. I didn't have a bike, so I was always on someone else's. They were in a shed. If the owner wasn't on duty you could take the bike. You put your bag on the back and cycled quite happily from Motherwell to Wishaw.

These were happy days. We weren't there for the money or the luxury or anything else but to be of service to humanity and we got on with it. Although we were deprived many a time, there was fun and jokes and I never worked with anybody spiteful. We'd plenty to say about the starchy sisters and all the rest of it, until I became one myself. But our own crowd, well we were all Jock Tamson's bairns. We couldn't compete with each other because we didn't have anything. Few of us had help from home. My sister sent me parcels but I'd no back-up as far as money went. Nobody was rich but we shared what we had – even cigarettes. Sometimes the patients would give you them and if anybody got a present of a packet they shared them out. A lot of us smoked in those days. We'd a big recreation room, a lovely room. Down the corridor was the smoke room. I hardly ever saw more than two people in the recreation room but in the smoke room it was standing room only.

We were expected to wear black stockings. In those days Woolworths was a thruppeny and sixpenny store. You could buy one stocking for sixpence. So, when we had a sixpence we could buy a stocking and hope that the other one wouldn't wear out. Of course they weren't silk stockings. They were either wool or cotton or lisle.

Sometimes we'd to go out on a dark night. There were no street-lamps because of the blackout. Not even lights from windoows because windows had all to be screened. We were provided with torches but as we had to have three thicknesses of tissue paper over the beam we finished up with a very faint light and it wasn't easy looking for the number of the house or the street. We poked this very poor light into nearly every door we came to, till we found the right one. If a policeman saw you doing that he'd come and help right away and take you to where you wanted to be. There were far more police-men on the beat then compared to now. They didn't race about in cars. They were there and ready to help.

Even in the very rough districts we went without fear of being molested. If they saw the little black bag, that was your defence against any kind of hooliganism. In their own way they respected us.

Lighting in houses was mostly gas mantles. In the blackout we never knew when the air-raid warden was going to come and knock on the window and say there was a light shining – the least chink of light showing at the side. All the windows had special frames made for them.

At Motherwell we didn't take out medical students as they did in Rotten Row. Motherwell was a midwifery training school only. We'd doctor there, a woman. There'd been a man doctor but he was away at the war. This woman was very nice and very able. She lived out, so at night time there was only a midwife there all night and if we needed the doctor for forceps or a Caesarean section we'd phone for her. There was an anaesthetist who would come but quite often a midwifery sister gave the anaesthetic. They started off with chloroform and there was a machine that kept the anaesthesia going. Now you have an injection in your arm and you don't know a thing. They didn't seem to do a lot of sections. I reckon if any case in Motherwell was considered to be very difficult the mother was sent to Rotten Row.

Yet I delivered triplets without any bother at Motherwell and I had twins there as well. They're in my Blue Book of cases. When it was completed, was sent in to the examiners and you could be questioned on it but I was lucky. I think they thought it was quite well done. The Final was held in Stobhill in Glasgow. I was allocated a patient for my exam and she must have thought I was a doctor. We had to stand beside who we had been allocated, and she started telling me all about herself. After that I could answer all the examiners' questions without any bother at all.

Ella Banks and Linda Stamp

It was a fulfilling job. I made a lot of friends some of whom are dead and gone but some like Linda who I still keep up with. It's good to have her near. I was the Matron here and when I got married she came up and took the job here. She had to work her notice and my husband allowed me to work for a month till Linda came up. That was a great concession. Wives were supposed to be at home then. Wives *were* at home then. She was the right Matron for the job. I just wore a white cap with a frill round it but she wore an Army square and her navy blue dress with the white collar. She was every bit the Matron.

The first delivery I ever saw as I told you was that posthumous one. One of my last deliveries, the doctor told me, 'You'll never see this again I hope'. It was a mermaid baby. It had its face and its head and it had arms but its legs were joined right down and its feet. It died of course. It was very very deformed. I didn't see many others deformed.

There wasn't much instruction to the mothers as far as bathing went. On the District they liked to watch us bathing the baby but they didn't get to watch in hospital. They did get to handle their babies at feeding time but then they were taken from them back to the nursery till the next feeding time. Even when the fathers wanted to see their baby they were taken to look in the nursery.

The babies were lovely. We grew so fond of them, we could hardly part with them. In the nursery we bathed them in the morning and we'd say, 'I'm doing Baby So-and-So.' We all had our favourites. Some of them you could make to look so lovely. Some had a lot of hair and some were almost bald and the ones with a lot of hair you could make into a nice cock's comb which at the time was very much the fashion for babies' hair. The poor little baldies. But we loved them all.

12

PEGGY GRIEVE

*After training as a midwife in Glasgow Maternity Hospital,
Peggy Grieve worked as a midwife, first at Cresswell Hospital
Dumfries, where she was a Staff Midwife, Sister Midwife and
Midwifery Tutor before moving to Fife to be Head of Midwifery there. She was also on the Central Midwives' Board for
Scotland for a time. She has been a member of the Royal
College of Midwives since 1948 and played an active part as
chairman of Scottish Board, member of the RCM Council and
chairman of the Executive Committee. In retirement, she still
takes a lively interest in the RCM Scottish Board. She now
lives in Lockerbie.*

I started midwifery training in January 1946 at the Royal
Maternity Hospital in Glasgow having previously done general nurse training. At that time midwifery training was in
two parts. Part 1 was mainly theoretical and Part 2 was
mostly clinical experience. In Part 1 we had to have ten
deliveries. We had experience in antenatal and postnatal but
no formal teaching in either and no clinics. We had a lecture
every day usually at nine o' clock in the morning with an
occasional evening lecture which was much better for those
on night duty. On day duty, if you were off duty you could go.
If you were on duty, you could go if the ward was quiet. We
had exams after each Part. Part 1 was written and clinical,
and Part 2 – we wrote up a blue Case Book for the twenty
statutory deliveries and also had an oral exam.

In Part 2 to begin with I went to the labour ward for about
ten days and I had two deliveries and then I went on the
District. Student midwives went out on their own and sometimes with a medical student. I can always remember the

ladies saying to me, 'We like the maternity nurses, [Rotten Row pupil midwives] we dinna like the Green Ladies.'Of course we knew why they didn't like the Green Ladies. It was because they were trained. We weren't, and we were frightened to tell them what to do.

The husband had to come to the hospital for us and we would go by tram. If it was during the night from 11 p.m. to 6a.m., we walked – to Maryhill, Denniston . we got to know Glasgow very well. When we did follow up visits we got tokens for the trams. One Saturday afternoon, I had a list of visits and I was standing at Glasgow Cross waiting for a tram. A football match was on and the men were waiting for the tram which was loaded. The clippie put out her hand and said, 'The nurse only.' The order to 'make yourselves prominent,' worked.

If you didn't get to the place on time it was a BBA which was 'Born Before Arrival' and that didn't count as a delivery. I had a terrible spell of about six or seven BBAs. So I was put on call first every night sometimes going out twice in a night. One night I'd had a BBA and I was called again about five a.m. The father was waiting to escort me to the Gallowgate. He told me that they already had twelve children, all alive and under fourteen. All went well with the delivery. We had no ergometrine for the third stage, only oral liquid ergot which we were only supposed to give if the mother was bleeding. I gave it prophylactically – particularly in that case.

The admission room at Rotten Row was known as the 'slab'with a tartar of a midwife in charge, often with a student. Patients, some with no antenatal care, some very poor would arrive there. They were stripped of their clothes and whoever was with them would take them home. They were washed and put into hospital gowns that opened down the back. They had red dressing gowns and a red cape for sitting up in bed. Before they went home they were taken down to outpatients and the nightie was taken off them before they went home.

It was called the slab because there was a slab of formica like a work surface and the mothers were literally put on it. It was a square room with two slabs each covered with only a sheet. They used to whip the sheet off if somebody came in pretty dirty. There was always a doctor on admission to see them and he was probably on call for the labour ward as well. These mothers were coming in in labour. Even if they came in pushing they didn't bypass the slab. Sometimes they even delivered there.

Cresswell, Dumfries

After I passed I went to Cresswell Maternity Hospital which was created from the local Poor House at the beginning of the war for pregnant women evacuated from Glasgow. The small maternity home already in the town was not big enough. Dr Bruce Dewar, later a Chairman of the Central Midwives Board for Scotland, was sent from Edinburgh to organise obstetrics there. At that time there were eighty beds on two floors, the bottom for non-private patients, the top for private patients. The non-private patient, making up about two thirds of the total, paid £5 for the time she was in regardless of how long it was. The private patients paid about £9, £8, or £7 a week for a single, double or three or four bedded room respectively. Sometimes they were in longer than the planned fortnight and they became very anxious about their finances. Some bills could be adjusted but it was never straightforward. If their husbands were insured they got a grant of about £2 but if they came into hospital they didn't get the Maternity Grant. When the National Health Service started in 1948 everyone came in free. There was no difference in the care but in the private ward they had an individual teapot on their tray.

Staffing levels were low. There were about eighty deliveries in the month at that time. After I had been there about six months and had some labour ward experience I was put on night duty. There was a night sister, a staff midwife which was me, two students and two auxiliaries. One night I was told that the sister was off sick and I was in charge of the hospital.

Peggy Grieve

A husband phoned the antenatal ward, from the Mull of Galloway, enquiring after his wife. I had to look through the book because I didn't know them. She was about forty-five, having her eighth child and in with hypertension. Her blood pressure had settled and I told him she was satisfactory and he said, 'Can I inquire for somebody else?' and I said, 'Is she a friend?' He said, 'She's my daughter.' The mother was having this one and the daughter was having her first one . . . He cycled two miles every night about half past nine to inquire on the phone for his wife and we got to know each other quite well. I would say to her, 'Your husband phoned.' 'Ask him how the bairns are.' I said to the man, 'I've to ask about the bairns.' 'Tell her they're all fine. So-and-so is looking after the house and she's doing very well. The others are going to school and the wee one is with her mother and he's all right.' There was the husband keeping that home together with the second-oldest daughter off school to run the house and the young one with his granny. One Friday night he said, 'Tell my daughter her husband will be up on Saturday at visiting time.' and I said to him, 'Are you no coming?' He said, 'I havena the money tae come wi.' I said, 'I'm sorry, but anyway I'll give them your message.' I didn't say to his wife that he hadn't the money. Working on the farms he was probably getting about a couple of pounds a week.

We saw lots of complications including severe pre-eclampsia and eclampsia. Dr Bruce Dewar had worked with Professor Morris who was obstetrician in charge of Irvine Maternity Hospital, in Ayrshire. They started treating eclampsias with tribromethanol which worked very well. These patients used to be completely unconscious probably for three days – these were the eclamptics and if it was severe pre-eclampsia they probably put them under too. It was given rectally and supposed to be according to the weight of the patient. You couldn't assess this if the patient was in a convulsion so they took the average weight of a woman and gave the dose accordingly. So the smaller ones stayed under longer with their first dose while the bigger ones needed another dose more quickly. Severe pre-eclamptics were sectioned like that – put under and then taken, given a general anaesthetic and sectioned and you got a live child and mother. We also saw concealed accidental haemorrhage, placenta praevias and severe anaemia, particularly folic acid deficiency anaemia.

At that time the GPs did the antenatal care although some clinics were at the hospital. Women were away from home for hours for a clinic visit. One woman left her home in the Thornhill area at 8.30 a.m. to get a bus to Thornhill, then toDumfries and from the town centre up to Cresswell for the clinic and then back. By the time she got home it would almost 6 p.m. I'm sure the public transport isn't any better in that area today.

After that, more obstetric staff came and they started peripheral antenatal clinics in Langholm, Annan, Castle Douglas, Kirkcudbright, Newton Stewart, Stranraer and Kirkconnel. The doctors went out to these clinics but they were run by domiciliary midwives. Often they were treble-duty staff in those areas.

Dr Bruce Dewar, was superb. He would come along on his own and ask how things were. If you got the junior, it was my job to guide them. Some of them accepted it quite well and others objected and could be quite obstructive if you suggested what a mother should have for sedation. I used to get Bruce Dewar to have a word with them.

Sometimes there was a complication at home known as 'failed forceps'. I remember the first one I saw. I said, 'Failed forceps?' Bruce Dewar said, 'Yes.' The GP phoned at about six p.m. He said, 'You always got them about six pm or early, about eight o'clock in the morning.' What happened was, the GP had been with the patient, he had a surgery waiting for him, and to get the baby delivered, he would apply the forceps. Quite probably there was a rim of cervix and he couldn't manage to deliver the baby. Then of course the mother was admitted. Very often they had a constriction ring, Bandl's ring. On the anaesthetic trolley we always had ampoules of amyl nitrite. So they had to have deep anaesthetic with amyl nitrite which released the ring when it was inhaled. People also used it for angina in those days. It was in a glass capsule which you broke, you put it in a swab and put it under their noses. Sometimes they had two. Usually they did an examination under anaesthetic and if a vaginal delivery was not possible, they did a Caesarean Section.

As far as failed forceps was concerned, the GP had a problem. He had probably sat with the patient and the midwife a few hours. He knew he had a surgery full of patients waiting for him. I can remember five or six failed forceps in my time. There were also patients having a home confinement. They came in exhausted and dehydrated because they had been in labour for up to forty-eight hours. All these patients had a GP booked and even though it was part of their job, a lot depended on how efficient and keen the GP was to do midwifery. The midwife could attend the confinement and be on her own and be in charge but if there were any complications she had to get the GP.

Cresswell was very primitive because it had started as a poorhouse. They gradually adjusted and extended it until the 1960s when there would have been about eighty beds and twenty premature cots.

It had a big area to cover and the Flying Squad covered Dumfries. We got delayed labours, PPHs, retained placentas. We had everything ready and drums which we took with us.Going out with the Flying Squad would be the obstetrician, probably the registrar, a staff midwife or a sister and probably a student. We didn't send a paediatrician because we only had one. One time, in the 1950s, I was sent out with the ambulance because they had phoned to say there was a patient having an abortion. When we got there we couldn't move her. She was lying, white, in a pool of blood. I could see her chamber under the bed and it was half full of clotted blood. I asked the ambulance driver to phone the hospital and ask if the flying squad would come. We put the end of her bed up on blocks. Frank Shaw came out in his car with O-negative blood and the equipment because we had the ambulance there. We had a little centrifuge where you cawed the handle to cross-match the blood. We put her on blood in the house.

Another patient in labour up New Galloway way phoned in a terrible snowstorm wanting the ambulance. The husband walked so many miles from the gamekeeper's cottage and they had the snow ploughs out and we followed the snow plough up to the house. We got up and got her loaded. The snow was very deep round the house and they had to do a lot of digging before they got the ambulance turned and away. That was in the days when snow was snow.

There were many more stillbirths than there are now and I don't think there was the psychological trauma then – not the same as it is today. I have heard the obstetrician say, 'Now don't worry, you can have another baby next year.' Now, the trauma is very much bigger because of the smaller number of children and also their expectations are different.

Very small premature babies did not live and we had very little to help them with. I can remember giving oxygen with a little funnel just lying beside the baby. We had little wooden boxes made by the joiner and they had the lining with little pockets all round and we put hot water bottles all round the baby. You re-filled them hourly in rotation. There was no special nursery for them. There was a smaller room but it was often used for babies with an infection.

As time went on there was family planning. I can remember mothers of forty plus coming in and probably having up to ten babies. If it was an emergency, they were always so afraid of the hospital. They had never been in hospital. I remember one woman saying to me,'Am I going to die?' I said,' No, of course you're not going to die.' She said,'I don't care but I think about the bairns.' They all had this in their minds.

I used to say to Bruce Dewar,' Are you going to sterilise her?' 'How can I sterilise her? I haven't got the husband's permission.' I said,'The husband's permission!' We used to try and get it. This husband phoned up and I said to him 'In the operation would you agree that Doctor sterilises your wife?' He said, 'Oh, aye.' I said, 'Well you'll need to come in tonight and sign a form.' I said this to Bruce Dewar and he said, 'On your head be it if you don't get the form!' Well she was sterilised and the form was signed. He used to say,'I could lose my livlihood for this.' The woman agreed – she was desperate to be sterilised but you still had to get the husband's permission at that time.

He came in one day and he said, 'There's something for you. Read that. That's the answer to your big families.' It was about the Pill. That must have been in the late fifties, or beginning sixties just before it started and it was the Report of the trial runs in Puerto Rico. There had also been a successful short trial in Manchester then it started from there.

I was a sister by that time and of course the staff had increased. Cresswell became a Part 1 midwifery training school in about 1944 and then it became a Part 2 plus Part 1 about 1956. I started my Midwife Teachers' Diploma (MTD). They have me a day release a week to Edinburgh and I travelled to the Simpson. I had to pay for my fare, my books and so on. There was a probationary period of six weeks, then an oral and written entrance exam and then Parts 1 and 2.

I qualified in 1956, still on the staff at Cresswell. The new hospital had been built and I became labour ward superintendent. Departmental sister – the best job I ever had. I don't think I would have left it but it was strenuous and I felt I would never maintain the pace till I was sixty. A teaching post came up in 1962 which I applied for and I became a tutor. I taught on the clinical side while I was labour ward superintendent. It was wonderful because you were teaching and relating to the classroom. It was difficult standing back at times. The midwives would come and say, 'What will I do?' I would say, 'If I weren't here, what would you do?' That got them to take responsibility.

We started a package system, for autoclaving instruments. After that it became divisional but we started it in Cresswell. If you had an emergency section or a prolapse of the cord they wanted to do it immediately. If electric sterilisers went off the boil they took some time before they came back to the boil again and really held things up in an emergency. I said, 'We're going to try autoclaving out.' We did it and it was good.

So I went to the classroom as a tutor. By this time we had

about thirty student midwives with four intakes a year. Also, the student nurses had to have experience. So they employed another tutor and I was the senior tutor.

Then the Salmon structure came in and my grade was only at the grade of nursing officer. This was because it was not a big enough hospital for the senior person to be a principal nursing officer. I went to the College and the Scottish Home and Health Department but got nowhere. I applied for a job at Stobhill in Glasgow but I fell out with the obstetrician at the interview. He and I just didn't see eye to eye. I became a bit discouraged and did not want to apply for anything else. However, Miss Becket, Education Officer for the Central Midwives Board phoned me and said, 'Fife's coming up. Get applying.' At that time it was Forth Park, Craigtoun at St Andrew's, and Newport. I got the job and I went to Fife.

This was in the 1970s. In the time I was at Cresswell deliveries had gone from eighty to two hundred a month. In that time we started parentcraft and family planning. It was one of the first areas that had 100% hospital confinement because Bruce Dewar was all for hospital confinement. He had a very good relationship with the district nurses and GPs.

I came to Fife as Principal Nursing Officer in Charge of Midwifery and Dr Melville who was MOH in Kirkcaldy had approached Forth Park about integration of community midwifery in Kirkcaldy. There were no (or few) home confinements but there was postnatal care. They granted me money for a full-time and a part-time midwife and that was integration started in Kirkcaldy. Then Dr Riddle who was MOH in Fife County came to negotiate. They could not give any money for staff so we had to get it through the Hospital Board. So we took over Glenrothes, then the district between Glenrothes and Kirkcaldy. We also did Burntisland, Auchtertool and Puddledub which was East Fife. Then we took over North East Fife planning to start on 1st June and it was snowing. The last place was Leven and around there. As integration happened, we offered the GPs a midwife to go to their antenatal clinics. I went to the GPs and said, 'Now she's coming to your clinic but I don't expect her just to to take blood pressures and test urines. She's there as a midwife and she should examine some of your patients.' They were also expected to give advice to the mothers on health issues and things like that. One GP was not very happy at the outset and I reminded him of the statutory ruling of the CMB which said that mothers should be seen by a practising midwife post-natally for ten days and this was not happening. Anyway, we started it and I met him sometime later. He said, 'That was a great invention.' Integration worked well in Fife.

We also had parentcraft going on everywhere and family planning nurses coming into the hospital. They used to come in once a week and then we got a liaison health visitor who worked between the hospital and the outside. That was very good because she came across family and domestic problems.

The new hospital was planned. The first part was opened in Kirkcaldy, at Forth Park, and the second bit was just started. The old house was used, but there was the antenatal ward in Forth Park and then there were five delivery rooms below it. It was planned as a GP unit, and then the GPs didn't want it. By this time Dr Duthie was here and he wanted a proper obstetric unit. The birth rate was still going up and they planned the extension. The foundations were started when I arrived. They had problems with the foundations because of all the mining in Fife and they had to grout very carefully. It took a long while.

Craigtoun was a lovely mansion house with beautiful cornicing and staircase still with its red carpet. The staff were very loyal but sadly it was not ideal for an obstetric hospital and it had to close. There was also a small GP unit at Newport. The local people were not happy at losing their maternity unit at Craigtoun and there were many meetings which eventually resulted in Craigtoun closing for deliveries. We transferred mothers to Forth Park for delivery and returned them to Craigtoun for postnatal care. That carried on for some time and then it closed altogether. Also, as the new hospital was opening, the two consultant paediatricians, one appointed the same time as I was, wanted to do intensive care of the neonate so we had send staff away to train for that. There was also the labour ward intensive care. We had to get more tutors and we also had a clinical tutor to teach in the clinical area. We were well staffed and we had full integration.

We had a good relationship with GPs and other doctors. There was only one doctor with whom I had no relationship. He was offensive to the midwives to the point of reducing them to tears and I refused to stand it. I put in a formal complaint about him and after a final set-to with him in my office the bullying stopped. I was not used to having trouble with doctors. I remember this doctor saying to me before he went out of the office that day, 'I think we could work together.' I said, 'Yes, we could work together, Doctor, not for you. I've worked with a lot of doctors but with them, not for them.'

In the training of the student midwives we always emphasised the relationship of theory to clinical practice. It was excellent to have the clinical tutor. They help to emphasise the important relationship between the theory and the clinical practice. The hours of clinical experience are essential, as essential as theoretical training. Possibly the clinical experience is not given the same emphasis now.

13

ANNE BAYNE

Anne had a lifelong ambition to be a district nurse and have a little car like the district nurse she knew as a child in Aberdeenshire. This involved nurse training, midwifery training and Queen's Nurse training before being allowed to practise as a district nurse/midwife in Clackmannanshire. Anne's story here covers midwifery training at Lennox Castle Hospital, life as a Queen's Nurse, and then as a midwife and clinical teacher in midwifery in Stirling.

One: Midwifery Training

When I finished my nursing training in Aberdeen Royal in 1951, I wanted to do midwifery. At that time the training was in two Parts. Part 1 allowed you to be a maternity nurse and Part 2 certified you as a midwife. As there was a shortage of places in Aberdeen for Part 2, many girls only did Part 1 there. My friend and I wanted to do both parts in one place and were accepted to do this at Lennox Castle starting at the end of 1951.

It was a huge cultural shock. We came from sheltered lives in the depths of the country in north-east Scotland. Aberdeen was our metropolis, and to come to Lennox Castle, just seventeen miles out of Glasgow, was a huge eye-opener.

It had been a large mental hospital for a long time. When war came a part of it was taken over by the Department of Health for Scotland as an emergency maternity home. There were three units each having two big wards, a couple of smaller wards, a kitchen and a huge antiquated bathroom with a bath in the middle of the floor. Each ward had eighteen beds up the sides with a sluice with bedpans at the end. There was a dining room and three huts for our use – a teaching hut, matron's office and the administrative offices.

Mothers from Glasgow came to Lennox Castle. Poor things. Many of them lived in Gorbals tenements. Most of them had head lice and didn't seem to worry about it – it it was just part of their condition. If you had one person who was clean, the others would borrow her comb so she ended up with head lice too. I had seldom seen head lice before – it was thought to be terrible. Some also had pubic lice.

There was very little to work with at Lennox Castle. They were given what you might call battlefield equipment and made a maternity hospital out of nothing. We made our cord-ligatures ourselves with cotton and forceps. We were dab hands at it. Then you put it into the spirit to sterilise it and that was your cord ligature made.

After we delivered the women they had to stay seven or eight days. A bus came at eleven o'clock to take them back into Glasgow when they were discharged. We had a funny old sister and an assistant sister who was an old dear. She used to colour her hair and she used to spray her hair and her specs with tinsel. All she did was the crossword. You didn't interrupt her until she had completed this. The old postnatal sister, would be shouting 'Where is she?' and she would hide and say, 'I haven't finished the crossword yet'. She also did the 'OR book'. She went round and she would say,'When did you have your baby? Oh, three days ago. Well is it no' time you should be back to your man?' 'Oh, I don't . . .' 'Well sign the book here and you can go hame the morn'. That was OR – Own Request. This was how she got rid of them. If they signed that book they could go. She couldn't stand them lying there being attended to.

A lot of the mothers came out to Lennox Castle and Tweedie Brown, one of the consultants, used to see them at the clinic. They travelled by bus from Dundas Street, Glasgow and walked about half a mile up the avenue. We also had a clinic in Glasgow at Montrose Street on one afternoon a week. You would set up the things for the clinic and by the time you had set it up it was all covered with smuts.

Anne Bayne

One day a young lass expecting her first baby went in and she saw Tweedie Brown. He examined her and said, 'Well lass, I'm afraid the baby has died. Now you'll just need to go home and wait and when you go into labour, come back in'. And out she went. I was really worried about her. This young lass would need to get the bus back into Dundas Street and then she would likely have to get another bus to go somewhere else probably by herself . . . I got her dressed and there was another woman who was expecting baby number three or four. I asked her if she was going back to Glasgow. When she said, 'Yes', I said to her, 'Do you see that lass there? Could you take her under your wing? She's had some bad news which I don't think has sunk in and I don't know if her husband is going to be at Dundas Street to meet her'. She said, 'Dinna you worry nurse, I'll look efter her'. Away they went.

They didn't induce labour for that at that time. She had to wait until she went into labour and she had her stillborn baby. It was a shame but that was the norm then along with high parities; eight, nine, ten babies was quite usual.

We had a first stage room with four army camp beds. The women in labour lay there and we pulled the screens across between them. I can still see one Irish girl who had been a nun and had come to do midwifery before going back to the convent. She was big-built and as Irish as could be and she was always knitting. She would say, 'Just breathe in and out dear, breathe in and out'. She had this row of pattern to finish before she could go and see to the patient.

Lennox Castle was used in a way like an overflow. It stayed in operation until the Queen Mother's Hospital was opened around 1964 and was then handed back to the mental hospital. Our matron was Miss Weatherburn, a very tall thin lady. She was tremendous. She was also our tutor and a great teacher. She was the one that first sowed the seeds in me to go into teaching. She wanted me to stay on and staff, saying, 'If you do, I'll give you classes to take'. But at that stage, I still had this dream of this little car and I thought, 'No I want to do district nursing'.

I had about a hundred deliveries in Part 1. Then out on

Scottish Midwives

community in Part 2; you always got your ten deliveries on community. A lot of girls who had been at Aberdeen with me came to do Part 2. At one time we had more Aberdonians there than anyone else and we got tremendous experience which was great for when we went out on district. Montrose Street was the headquarters where we met for community. We walked down to the bus and got the bus in in the morning, went to Montrose Street and you were given your list of where you had to go. If somebody was in labour and you were needing the deliveries you waited to do the deliveries.

Some of the houses were just unbelievable. There was one house just right across from Duke Street prison. We went up into this room. There was only one decent chair. The other chair was an old fashioned kitchen chair with a round seat, only there was no bottom in it. There was just the rim. We couldn't decide whether it was safer to sit on this rim or sit in the other chair, because of the fleas. We lived our lives with fleas. We got a chemist to mix DDT with our talcum powder to try and control them because I used to come up in great welts with the bites. Montrose Street itself was just hotching. We dusted everything we could with this DDT-talcum powder to try and keep the fleas at bay. The community midwife, who was a Green Lady, and I sat with this mother. That was the day we had had a cup of tea and then the little fellow, the older brother, appeared and he used the teapot to pass urine in. We didn't need to have a delicate constitution.

When the Queen's Nurses in Glasgow booked a mother they laid down very strict rules. The Green Ladies made no demands. So, working with the Green Ladies, we went into the poorer houses and worked with what was there and sometimes it was precious little. That was one that I remember and we took turn about in this chair till the baby was delivered.

Night duty was where we got most of our experience. A taxi would be phoned for and would come for us. One night I was sent for and the Green Lady was late. The address was in Nicholson Street. This street was to me, a stranger in the place, almost the pits. I think Nicholson Street had probably

96

been one of these marvellous Edwardian mansion streets that were established with the shipbuilding trades. Now it was all let and whole families lived in one room. There would probably be one shared toilet and there was usually one shared sink. On this occasion I got the address and I went up. I think their name was Singh and when I arrived there were many families called Singh there. I knocked on the door. The woman opened it. She wasn't pregnant. I went round the doors like this. This was me just a student. Eventually a door was answered by a lady who was pregnant so I tried to get in and she was saying, 'No, no, no'. So that wasn't right either. I kept going until at last I knocked on a door and an old body opened it. I went in and I could hear definite labour pain. There she was on the bed which was, as usual, in the corner. There was the most amazing mat on the floor. It had strange signs on it and round it were all these men. Their turbans were off and they all had long hair and they were praying. I stood at the door and looked and I thought, 'She's going to deliver'. So I thought, 'What do I do here? There's nobody saying 'excuse me' or anything else'. They must have known that I had come in. So I said to myself, 'Right, Anne, the shortest way between two points is a straight line', so I just went for it. I got half way across this mat and they whipped it from under me and I landed on my back with my feet up. One of them was leaning over me – I can see his long hair yet – and he was saying 'You damned, you go to hell. You damned, you go to hell.' Nobody else seemed to be speaking. I picked myself up with what dignity I could and I went across to her. She didn't speak. They all just stayed there. I thought, 'If anything goes wrong with this delivery, I'm for it'. Remember the Green Lady hadn't arrived. I prepared as best I could. I can't remember that much. A woman appeared at the door with water. They knew the drill. I delivered this baby. As soon as the baby was born, these men took him from me. I delivered the placenta, and it was at that point that the Green Lady appeared: 'Oh well that was a good job done'. And that was it. I came out of there shaking like a leaf. It wasn't until afterwards in the taxi going back that it really hit me just what had happened and what I had been through. The students didn't do the postnatal care in that situation and often when the Green Lady went she didn't get in. As far as I was concerned I had done the delivery and that was the last you would see till she was pregnant again.

We had to do case studies for our Blue Book and one in particular was again in Nicholson Street. Both the Green Lady and the doctor were there this time. I think this woman was para eleven. She had this one room. She was thrilled because they had the sink – the jaw-box – in the window. There was a fireplace with a mantlepiece and a little open fire – a range – where she did all her cooking. That night the older boy and the father went into the next room. There was a box bed in the room with a sheet over it. Behind the sheet there were five children of varying ages and so there were five little peep-holes in the sheet. There was the mother's bed and at the end there was a heap of coal and a cot and there were two in the cot. Then there was another cot like a Moses basket across at the other side. There was another bath there and the last baby was in it and now we were delivering the new one. There wasn't room for the doctor and the midwife and myself to stand and we took it in turns to sit on the bed. There was a wee paraffin lamp which was all the light we had and we took turns to hold that depending on who was doing what. We had a soup plate, and a Higginson's syringe. We gave the enema out of this plate, she returned it into the plate. I handed it out of the door and I don't know where it went, and the plate came back. I took the placenta into that plate and I bathed the baby in it. About four a.m. the Green Lady said, 'Now everything's done. I'll go and phone for your taxi'. By the time the taxi came, the mother had told me about how the midwife had been murdered on the stairs. They went again at ten o'clock to visit her and never got in. She never opened the door to anybody going back to see her.

I once went to do a delivery in the Castlemilk area which was just being built. I took the tram as far as I could and I had no idea about the streets. I said to this policeman on the beat, 'Excuse me, I've got this address'. He said, 'Oh come on, I'll

Anne Bayne

take you.' So he took me and we went into one of these new houses. There was coal in the bath, there were floorboards up and it was really rough. The woman was far on in labour as usual. I delivered her and no midwife appeared. The one consolation was, the policeman stood outside the door and I thought, 'That's fine, I've got protection'. He stood there all that time. We had to be there an hour afterwards so I suppose in total it was about three and a half hours. He saw me back to the tram and I said, 'Thank you very much. You'll never know how much it meant to me you staying there'. 'Oh', he said, 'Nurse, I didna stay over you. I couldn't have walked back through there myself. I would have needed two of us. We mustn't walk there alone so you were my protection.'

In the early fifties there were the razor gangs. I delivered one of their babies. They lived in a pre-fab, a lovely little house, and he was an awful nice laddie. I said, 'Why do you do it.' He said, 'Oh well, we dinna need the police force. We just sort things out amongst oorsels'. It was late in the evening and he said, 'I'll walk you back to the bus', because he knew we went up through Glasgow Green. We were walking along and I said to him, 'You know there's a crowd following'. 'I know,' he said. 'That's my gang. Two reasons they're there. I couldn't come back through myself, so they're walking with me so that when I put you on the bus I can come back. Another thing, if I stepped out of line with you they would have me'. Nurses had a great respect. Ministers and nurses could walk anywhere in Glasgow and no-one would touch them. Well, we got to the bus that night and he shook hands with me, thanked me, handed me my bag and put me on the bus. As he turned to walk away they all gave me a wave.

When we were on the community in Glasgow we still stayed at Lennox Castle. On night duty we took our food which was absolutely hopeless with us, maybe a boiled egg and a slice of bread. We depended on pupil midwives coming to the headquarters at Montrose Street from hospitals all over Glasgow. They had very good kitchens and they provided food for us. We didn't have money to buy extra food. Our pay was seven pounds fifty a month.

There were also the 'Snowdrops'. They were Rottenrow pupil midwives and they were snobbish little things. They wouldn't talk to any of the rest of us. We were lower than five eighths. One day, I was coming back on duty and a Snowdrop was breaking her heart. I asked her what was wrong and she said, 'I've just done a delivery and and,' she said (because normally they wouldn't speak to you or us to them), and I said, 'Well, what's wrong?' She said, 'We had to take the placenta back because we have to examine it with the tutor to see that it's OK, and,' she said, 'I've left mine on the bus in a National Dried Milk tin.' We got on the tram, went down to the depot and went in. I said, 'Excuse me, we're looking for a National Dried Milk tin.' 'Right,' said the man, 'What's in it?' So we had to tell him what was in the tin. When I came back my friends couldn't believe that I had helped a Snowdrop! Remember she wouldn't have been allowed to count the delivery if she hadn't brought the placenta back.

I remember women suffering from VD. We never wore gloves when we delivered. Women often waited until the last minute and came in in advanced labour. You'd be delivering this woman and then she would lift her head and say, 'Oh by the way I'm being treated for venereal disease'.

We also had to have clinic experience of sexually transmitted diseases and I used to attend the venereal disease clinic in Govan on Tuesdays. I hope God will forgive me but every Monday night I used to sincerely pray that I wouldn't waken up on Tuesday and if I did would I just be violently ill and not have to go because this Tuesday afternoon clinic nearly killed me. It was these tiny little children. Peter – I could have loved him to bits – was a wee lad. He would have been eight or nine. He came on a Tuesday and you had to give him this horrible injection. Then you gave him a sweetie – that put me off sweets. What a bribery. I used to think to myself, 'I won't give him the injection this week. I'll just give him the sweetie'. Then I used to pray that he wouldn't come. Doing that to him just tore me apart. But of course I always did give him the injection and gave him his sweeties. He had VD from his mum.

Anne Bayne

Then there was Annie, a great character. She had given up. She had given up going wi they sailors and she would come in to get her injection. One day I said, 'Oh Annie, I like your dress, it's very nice'. 'Meet me the nicht, nurse,' she said. 'Meet me the nicht. There's a grand boat in. You'll get a new frock, you'll get a new frock the nicht'. There she was, going to mend her ways but she was going to get a new frock and I would get one too. It was after the war and so many men came back with VD and their wives didn't know. It wisna natural for them to be parted six years, and so many of them had played ball away from home and VD was just rife. It really breaks my heart now when I think of all the work that was done and these clinics did a tremendous clean-up, and the government poured money in to try and control it. So that was all part of midwifery training.

After thirty-six weeks of pregnancy, you went in and collected your brown box. This was the delivery box and in it was waterproof paper, cotton wool, sanitary towels and so on – and a bottle of Dettol. Well, the Dettol in Glasgow was always white! 'We got it like that Nurse. That was how it came.' They had used the Dettol and filled it up with water and when you put water into Dettol it turns white. So that was life at Lennox Castle.

Two: Queen's Nurse

When I finished my training I went to do my Queen's in Edinburgh. The base was a big mansion house in Castle Terrace. My room was so small, you couldn't put two hands out. There was no heating and I took rheumatic fever and was quite ill for a couple of months. I wisna really cared for properly.

We were taught to drive a car at the same time and you got ten lessons. It was hard going, physically more than mentally. Just hell on wheels as one of our drivers told us. All you could think of was what was next to be done. My district was from the Donaldson School at Haymarket right out to the Zoo and I did all that down to Gorgie Road. I had a bicycle with nae brakes. The policeman stood at point duty at the Haymarket where the five roads meet. Whether he knew that I had nae brakes or if it was just 'Here comes the nurse', he always stopped the traffic to let me sail through. We were very poorly fed but we were a voluntary organisation and didn't get grants from the Government. The training for a Queen's Nurse took four months if you were a midwife. So I had three years general nursing, one year's midwifery and four months Queen's Nursing to learn how to be a district nurse.

I qualified as a Queen's Nurse in July 1953 – a couple of months late because of the rheumatic fever. Some girls had been sponsored by an employing authority but I decided against that. Because of this, my contract with the Queen's Nursing Institute said when I qualified I could be sent any-where in Scotland for a year. After that I could please myself.

I was sent to Clackmannanshire as Clackmannan Relief. This meant I was sent wherever there were nurses off. Four of us shared a big house in Alloa – the central point for the area which I didn't know at all. The first district I relieved was what they called the bottom end of Alloa – South Alloa. We took night about to be on call and on my first Tuesday, it was my turn. Somebody in labour rang and gave me the address. I left a message for the next on call who was visiting friends, saying that I had been called out and set off thinking I'd better find instructions as I had no idea where to go. The only person I had attended for the three or four nights was a lady on insulin. She had a boxer dog so I used to pull the door handle so that she wouldn't open the door, and shout through. She always wore little plimsolls and men's stock-ings. I shouted through, 'Mrs B., it's me.' When she opened the door I said, 'I've got an address here to go and deliver a baby'. She escorted me along the road and into the sleaziest pub I've ever seen, right on the shore. When she shouted, out came this little man with a big jersey, and the cap and the wellie boots. 'Come wi me,' he said. And God bless us, he took me into this boat and we crossed the Forth. I had my delivery bag with me as well. We went ashore and I went into a lovely home and delivered the baby. I was that thrilled wi everything, and then he took me back and I thanked him very much. I didna ken about payment but he wouldn't take anything.

I returned to the house where the other three were waiting. 'Where have ye been?' I said, 'I've been delivering a baby.' 'Where aboot.' 'In South Alloa.' 'South Alloa? That's no even our county. South Alloa is in Airth.' I was across the Forth in Airth. I said, 'Well that was the address they gave me'. 'How did you get there?' So I telt them. I had to fill out a form that I had practised outside my area. I wasna a week in the place and I was already rocking the boat. Dr Warren the assistant and Dr Borrowman the Medical Officer, they were not amused.

I really was too young and inexperienced then to cope wi these people. Brought up in a generation where we were seen and not heard, when people spoke to you you just accepted it. You never spoke back. They must have thought I was a twit and I was, probably, but that is where I lacked the maturity and this spoilt some of my enjoyment during these years. I just didn't know how to cope sometimes. I was twenty-three. After that experience which I never forgot they would say, 'Remember and stay in your own district'.

I also relieved in Alva and Menstrie but I was very ill in Alva when I was there because it was too near the hills and it didn't agree with my asthma. The doctor came down to see me and he said, 'Lassie, get oot o here. Ye'll need to go up the hill. Ye'll never ever live here'. There were many asthma patients in Alva because it was so near the hills.

The next place was Tullibody, as relief first, and when the Tullibody nurse left to get married, I got her post and lived there. It was a New Town. There was old Tullibody which consisted of a few streets, little old cottages and very much the little elite introverted mining village. Then a lot of new houses went up with the influx of miners from Lanark and Ayrshire bringing their own way of life which didn't go down well with the old folks in Tullibody.

It was a young population. Over the three years I was there until I married, I did an average of ten deliveries a month and interspersed with that I had total patient care. I had the old folks and I did dressings and I had the diabetics. It was a great way of life. These people too, being miners, in a way they were very protective of me. At one point the area was provided with a little Vespa scooter. They decided as I had a fairly big work-load, and as the rheumatic fever had left me with a slightly dicky valve in my heart, I should have the Vespa. The first night I had it Sandy vowed he was going to be a widower before he was even married. Nobody knew how to start it and I had some fun getting going. The Vespa took a gallon of a mixture of two-star petrol plus a pint of oil. Halfway along the road towards Stirling from Tullibody there was the Black Grange Petrol Pump. I went down to the man there and showed him the Vespa and this little booklet which told us the mixture. 'That's OK,' he said. 'We'll just get this wee drum.' He wrote NURSE in big writing on it. Then he said, 'Now, we'll measure in the gallon of petrol, add the oil and we'll gie it a good shak and we'll fill up your tank.' But my tank didna hold the gallon and the extra oil. 'Nobody will touch it and next time we'll do the same.' I got somewhere around 150 miles to the gallon. I had that Vespa for three years and I would say to the man, 'Now I need to pay my petrol bill.' He would say, 'Oh aye, aye, nurse, now I hinna ma books made oot. They're in the hoose, I'll get it again'. This went on and I never paid for petrol until it came to the time that I was getting married and I said to him one time I was in filling up, 'Now I must get this bill'. I hadn't a clue what it was going to come to by this time. At the same time, I said, 'I don't know what to do with the bike because they told me it was mine and I've had it all this time'. He said, 'Oh well, I ken somebody in the Health Board. You bring it doon tae me'. He found out what its price was and when I went back he said, 'Now nurse, your bill, I kent you werna runnin up a bill. He says yer bill's been peyed'. I got the cost price of the bike as well. So that's the sort of thing that went on. I've nae doubt that it was miners who did that. Also, I got an allowance of coal which usually was enough. Occasionally I went home and thought, 'I've mair coal than I had this morning'. Some of the miners would say to those who were delivering, 'Put some into the Nurse's'. They were very good to me. I stayed in the Nurse's lovely five-apartment house right opposite the church in Menstrie Road in Tullibody and used one of the rooms as a surgery.

At that time penicillin was the in thing. The miners would come in past, 'I've got a prescription for penicillin', and they would have six vials of penicillin, one for each day. I would give them the first one and the second the following day. By that time they were feeling better and tended not to return. I was left with the remaining vials of penicillin. I went to the chemist and said 'You know, I've got more penicillin in my house than you've got in your shop. What will I do with it?' 'Bring it back,' he said. So I did. Now he couldn't give this penicillin with the broken seal to anybody else. So he would say to the miner with a prescription, 'Go up and see Nurse Ramsay'. I don't know, we were maybe breaking the law but at least we werena wasting the penicillin. I thought, 'I canna pit it oot in the bucket'. I suppose legally he should have destroyed it but think of the waste and the money that it cost.

I averaged ten deliveries a month. The midwife who did the other half of the district was an 'old' resident and she was now married and lived in her own house. She didna like midwifery very much. So these young couples when they came to about thirty-six weeks moved into my district to stay with sisters or cousins and then I delivered them. They were there and I had to take them on.

One year when I came back from my Christmas break, for the next six weeks I never had a full night in my bed. We had half a day off a week and a weekend a month. The rest of the time I was on call and we just accepted it. You werena supposed to do midwifery *and* lay out bodies. Well, I did. They were people I had nursed. You couldn't say no to a request like that. You were often with them when they were dying; supported the family and became friends. It was a very special position you were in.

I got to know the people very well. I liked the family feel which gradually became less as different families flitted in. I usually saw my mothers who were due, in the morning just after I had done my insulins. I would see the mother and then I would knock on the lass's mother's door and ask if she was going to be in because her daughter could be doing with a visit. Or it could be an older sister or a cousin. The relatives were there for them. People didna have phones then. I used to leave addresses up on my door but more often I gave them to the people that were involved. They would say, 'Don't worry, Nurse, we'll keep an eye on things'. That's missing now.

I enjoyed my home confinements. I delivered two sets of twins at home and they should have been born in hospital which I would have preferred with twins. With the first set, the GP was too bloody-minded to agree wi me that it was twins. They were baith six pound odds and I nearly lost the second baby.

The second lot was probably quite unforgiveable. If we needed a doctor we had to work with whoever was on call. Some doctors were interested in midwifery and some didna want to know. Some liked to know after the baby was born because they went in and got £7 for this. We had this lady doctor who wasn't a bit interested. A lot of the women went to her because she was 'the lady doctor'. I used to go to see the mothers until they were six months and after that the doctor was supposed to go in. I would phone and say, 'Mrs. So-and-So'. 'Oh I just had her down in my books to go and see her.' That was always the story. This mother was expecting her fifth baby. She had had twins before and all along she kept saying to me, 'You know I'm haein twins. It's exactly the same as my last twins'. And I agreed wi her.

I informed the lady doctor who would not agree that it was twins. Time wore on and I still insisted that she was having twins and should be going into hospital and I wrote it in her notes. The doctor never went near her, and I could not admit the woman off my own bat. I couldn't even send for the Flying Squad on my own. I had to get a doctor to come. A doctor couldn't phone from the house and say, 'We need the Flying Squad'. He had to come down and say, 'Yes I have seen the patient', and then go back and phone for the Flying Squad.

Anne Bayne

One night, just after ten, I was called to the mother in labour with her twins. I delivered one, not bad. The second one was really struggling to breathe. It had the typical hollow on its chest as though the first baby's head had been lying on its chest. I couldn't get the baby to breathe and I couldn't get her to stop bleeding. I sent somebody running for the doctor – this lady doctor – and she didna come. There I am rubbing up the fundus to make the uterus contract with blood through the bed on to the floor and I am also trying to resuscitate this baby. She came after a good three-quarters of an hour. She came in and I can see her yet. She had the most beautiful ice-blue blouse on. 'What can I do here?' I said, 'The Flying Squad, we need the Flying Squad. *Now*'. It was another three-quarters of an hour before the Flying Squad appeared with Dr R. in charge. I told her the story. The baby went into the incubator and we had a nail up on the wall and started giving the mother intravenous plasma before moving her. In the middle of all this she said, 'Has anybody sent for the husband?' Well naebody had sent for the husband so Dr R. sent the GP. She phoned the pit to bring the husband up and they brought the wrong man up. The fellow they did bring up – he nearly died. By the time the husband arrived they were off in the ambulance.

What a night that was. I can see that front room yet. There was blood everywhere and the place looked as though a bomb had dropped on it. When the Flying Squad had gone away with the mother and her babies, the GP turned and said, 'Well there's nothing more I can do here', and away she went. I was left wi this blitz to tidy up. The baby died but we saved the mum. Even if they had been in hospital the baby might not have lived. We didna have the knowledge and the equipment that we have now. But the mother should never have been delivered at home. Dr R. blew the GP to hell, she really did. At one point she said to me, 'Why is she being delivered at home?' I said, 'I've been trying since she was four months when I knew it was twins to have her hospitalised. One, because of her age' – she was in her early forties by then – 'and two because I knew it was twins and I knew the family history. She had problems with the twins the last time'. That really was a heartbreak of a night.

It was shocking that a midwife couldn't call out a Flying Squad and a doctor couldn't phone from home without seeing the mother. He couldn't even on the midwife's say-so get the Flying Squad. One GP used to do it – he used to say, 'You're the bloody expert. You don't need me to come and stand and say yes'.

I had a lot of good times in Tullibody. The patients were great. I had to leave when I got married because they didn't allow married women as Queen's Nurses especially in the nurse's house. I had a friend in Tullibody whose twins I delivered. We were great pals and one night we were going out somewhere. We walked from her house up to mine and I was in my uniform and she said, 'The next time remind me I'll never walk up through Tullibody with you in uniform again'. Every scruffy little child came saying, 'There's my nurse'. 'And,' she said, 'They had nae socks and shoes. Some of them had nae pants on.' I said, 'Well, that's the houses that I go into most'. I had a great rapport with the folk there. It was a wonderful time.

Three: Stirling

If you thought of marriage you were out. You couldn't be a Queen's Midwife then. I had a break and came back into midwifery in 1964. By that time home confinements were nearly all gone. I used tell the students that home confinements went oot o the window when interior spring mattresses and fitted carpets came in. At that time if you bought one it was for a lifetime. You couldn't risk spoiling it. Before that you washed the lino. We covered the thin mattresses with rubber and newspaper and there wisna much damage done. You couldn't afford to replace expensive things. That was really partly when home confinements went out of fashion. I found that anyway. I used to say, 'Can I pull this carpet up?' You worried in case it got marked. Also, maybe nowadays they would sue you. That certainly hadn't come into the vocabulary in those days.

Anne Bayne

Huge strides were made in the sixties and from then on. So much happened in midwifery like the use of syntometrine and incubators – there were no high-tech incubators before then. Anti-D I think was the biggest thing. The first times we used it, we had to decide who was going to give it, or, spill it – this minute amount was so precious. That was in 1964-65. We could only give it to prims when they were delivered so that they could have a second healthy baby. Not to anyone else – it was so scarce. After that it seemed as though there was something new every week.

I was only part-time when I went to Stirling. This meant I couldn't get a sister's post and I was a staff midwife for many years. In 1973 my son was coming up for 16. I spoke to the Senior Midwife about being full-time and she offered me a sister's post in Special Baby Care.

The minute I came back full time, Forbes Walker, midwife teacher, wanted me to teach student midwives. I always was interested in teaching and she sussed that out very quickly when we were in the old unit in Stirling Royal Infirmary. That was before the new unit was established. It was where Ward 9 is now. We had our own theatre and our own labour wards and we had postnatal and prenatal. It ran at the same time as Airthrey Castle but they only did normal deliveries. We had the same consultants. Airthrey Castle was opened up when the War came. It really wasn't suitable – it's a lovely castle. The hall with the carvings on the walls and that staircase are quite beautiful. But the women walked from downstairs upstairs to be delivered. You couldn't put lifts in. So they only did normal deliveries. They would probably do a forceps delivery there but if there was surgery at all we had to go up with the Flying Squad and bring them down to the Unit. At that time they wanted Airthrey Castle for the University. That was really why we got the new maternity unit in Stirling.

There was a transitional time between closing the old unit and starting the new, and closing Airthrey Castle. I still carried on at the old unit at Stirling Royal Infirmary until the last patient left. We started off by taking across the postnatal staff. We delivered the mothers in the old Unit, kept them an hour and then transferred them to the new Unit. It took a while before all was sorted out. I stayed until the last, and then when I came across I did relief of every area until she put me into the nursery. I had a lot of experience with sick babies by this time working in the nursery in the old unit and was happy to be sister in the new.

After that, Forbes asked me if I would consider teaching. Mind you I suppose I took about a hundred pounds a month drop in wages because there was no unsocial hours in teaching and it was Monday to Friday. It meant Sandy and I could have some more time together, with weekends, so I said, 'Right I'll take it'.

In the Nursery the biggest thing was the first baby we ventilated. It was hand ventilation. Two paediatricians and a lab technician made up a Heath Robinson type of ventilator and we stood and hand pumped. One of the times I got someone to stand in for me I said, ' Now you watch that. If that dips below such and such, ring for help'. I came rushing home here. I had no transport at the time. I came home, peeled the tatties, put on the dinner, left them a note – working until ten o'clock tonight – and rushed back in and I don't think she had blinked. She didn't know anything about babies but she was game to sit there and she just watched this monitor. That was how we did it and that baby lived. That was really the beginning of the development of the Vicker's ventilators.

One of the first fluids we gave was called a Cockburn's cocktail, called after the doctor who invented it. John Higgins phoned and got him to dictate it over the phone and got the lab to make it up. They had a great respect for each other. That's all part of the development of the Special Care Baby Unit. We've come great strides since then. Before the incubators, it was the Charlotte top that we had. Our cots were swivel cots. They were made of a metal basket with a lining of very starched white material, and the Charlotte top was a perspex lid that you put on the cot. It had a little shelf inside. You put a wet nappy in there for humidity and it had the fitting for putting oxygen in and you would turn it on at two

Anne Bayne

litres! We nearly gave all these babies two litres of oxygen.
We didna ken that you should measure it a bit better than
that.

The very first incubator that came was big, round and
green. It came at five o'clock on a Friday night. The first baby
was a little Baby Reid and the mother was a tinker on the
road. I put the baby in and the baby changed colour so I took
the baby out. Then I put the baby back in and the baby
changed colour because this round perspex thing made things
look different. Anyhow came night time and I had to give the
Report. I told the night staff what to do and what Baby Reid
needed, and I went home. I never shut an eye all night. I kept
thinking, 'What if the baby's dead? What if it overheats?
What if . . . ?' I was so glad to get in the next Saturday
morning and find the baby still alive and kicking and still in
the incubator. They didna ken that the baby could be taken
out. I told them that the baby had to be nursed in there and
that was it. So that was the first one. That was in 1965. It took
up so much room. Then we got the other more modern ones
and the Sputnik one went up to Airthrey Castle. I called it the
Sputnik. What happened to it, I don't know if anybody quite
knew. It could have gone to a third-world country or it's
maybe in a museum somewhere. Then we had the hot and dry
thermometers that we used in the prem unit and they were for
topping up the humidity – we had to keep topping it up. The
sweat would run off us in that incubator room. We had the
little pipettes with a valve at one end and the teat at the other
to help these tiny little ones to feed. We also did tube feeding,
and any baby that twitched at all, you gave him chloral
hydrate. A teaspoonful of chloral hydrate. Aye – they slept
wonderfully.

Phototherapy came in when we were still in the old unit,
and again we had to use the premature nursery. The babies
were supposed to be under it for a week which they couldn't
stand because it was always accompanied by green loose
stools and very often vomiting. We didn't have the six hours
on and six hours off routine or twelve on and twelve off. We
gave it continuously at that time and although it was good,

111

we always felt that we had an ill baby when this was going on. It was introduced when we were still in the old unit – perhaps about 1967.

Third stage of labour

For us older midwives this complete change in the management of the third stage of labour was very difficult to accept. Up until then you didn't touch the cord. Now, to be taught that you had to deliberately pull on this cord was so different and frightening. We used to hope that the mother would give a cough so that she would deliver the placenta and we wouldn't have to pull. This was the start of active management of the third stage. Before this it had been passive management with maternal effort and probably bracing the fundus. We gave ergometrine when the placenta was delivered. This was done routinely. Then Syntometrine came in and it was given with the delivery of the anterior shoulder, and then you got on and delivered the placenta but with a time limit of seven minutes. That took a lot of mental readjustment. I'm not sure how much difference it made overall. There were mothers who got on and delivered their baby and there wasn't much blood. It was great probably for the midwives because we didn't need to stand and wait for an hour or so, which is what I sometimes had to do on district. I remember waiting till three o'clock in the afternoon because I couldna get the doctor to come, and then he came and he said, 'Oh I thought you would have had the placenta delivered'. So Syntometrine would have been good for that. Also, there was the saving time and therefore saving money aspect. I couldn't always help but think that the saving of money in the time factor had as much to do with Syntometrine as it had with the mother.

The next thing that happened was the introduction of the Ventouse Extraction. One of the doctors – Dr Choudrey the registrar – was allowed to buy the equipment and he did the first Ventouse Extraction. Dr R. didn't attend and then later she asked me to demonstrate how to put it together. I had an awful job trying to fix it up, using the hand pump. I always admired those Indian or Egyptian men doing it. They had the technique for doing ventouse that we didn't have. They just seemed to know exactly when to put it on and they always did so well. So that was another thing that was introduced, and here we were wondering what was going to happen next.

In the bad old days we used to give oil, baths and enemas (OBE), and Dr R. used to look at us old timers and say there was nobody could give the OBE quite like us. Then they started using Buccal Pitocin. What a nightmare it was getting the women to suck all that. They would get to the second tablet and if it was going to work it would work. If not you could have sucked the whole lot and it wouldna work.

Then we went through the phase of episiotomy. It was maybe good in that we were controlling the perineal tear and it might be much easier sutured. However, at the same time women became far healthier, far more health-conscious, and so therefore they probably didn't need this intervention quite the same. I think each case should be taken on its own merits. I could see good in it but I could also see that we sometimes did it far too quickly. You've also got to take the expertise of the suturer into consideration as well.

Male midwives

Training of men to be midwives started in the late 1970s. Two hospitals in Britain were chosen to be pilots for this, one in London, and we were the Scottish pilot. The big difference that we made was, there was to be no chaperoning. *They* chaperoned their male midwives. Our reasoning was it would take away from our students' expertise if they were chaperoned and they would never become proficient practitioners in their own right. The good thing was that we had Annie Grant as our education officer at the CMB. She was tremendous. To me part of midwifery died when Annie Grant retired. If ever there was somebody who was 110% a midwife, it was Annie. She fought for us in Brussels, and she was adamant when we were changing the programme and the length of the programme that it should be right. She had very high standards. Anyhow – they (the English) chaperoned. We didn't. As she said, 'Any patient can refuse any member of staff male or female'. They can say, 'No I do not want . . . to deliver me'. That's their prerogative. She said, 'They can exercise those rights'. We never had any problem. In fact when we asked the mothers, they found the men very caring, often more so in lots of ways than the others.

When I was four my mother took me to visit my aunt in hospital in Aberdeen at Woolmanhill. This was in the 1930s and hospitals were kept up by voluntary donations. The nurse went round at visiting time with the plate. I had a white fur jacket and leggings and a little bonnet and they came and handed me the plate to take round the ward. As I did this, I thought, 'This is where I belong'. Things have moved a long way from then and from when I idolised the district nurse/midwife with her little car.

14

ELLA CLELLAND

Ella Clelland did midwifery training at Glasgow Royal Maternity Hospital and qualified in 1958. From there she practised as a midwife in Haddington where she saw a very different way of life. After a time practising in England, Ella returned to Scotland and became the District Nurse/Midwife for Callander and the Trossachs until she retired.

After my general training in Edinburgh I started midwifery in 1957 when it was still in two Parts. It was the done thing to train at the Simpson or Glasgow Rotten Row. The girls at the Simpson were always talking about 'We at the Simpson' and the Simpson 'ladies' and the Rotten Row 'midwives'. There was a huge waiting list for Rotten Row but I wanted desperately to train there as they had a wide spectrum of the abnormal and I wanted to gain experience in this. Glasgow people were always known to be smaller in stature. They had rickety children because of their poor diet and they had no sunshine coming into the tenement buildings and many mothers had rickety abnormal pelves. I did a year's staffing in Casualty with my name on the Rotten Row waiting list. I wrote to Rotten Row again and after about four months I was accepted.

I started there in September 1957 and hated the first six months. It was so intense you felt you were getting nowhere. There were medical students as well, so you had almost shared training with the medical students. Those days lectures were ongoing and it didn't matter if it was your day off – you had to stay and have your lecture. Duties started at 8am off at 12 pm, back at 4 pm till 9 pm. It was a pretty exhausting pace.

You had your stint in labour room. Labour rooms now look like somebody's front room compared to what they were like. In one room, we had six iron labour beds which didn't come apart like today's ones. This was not only a first-stage room. It was an every-stage room. The gas and air machines were wooden box affairs and made a lot of noise with these valves. You would hear the valves, all the pushing and shoving and oohing and aahing and lots of midwives dishing out instructions. We said it was like Waverley Station – it was really quite bizarre.

Even although you had the advantage of anatomy and physiology from general training, it was very intense. We felt we couldn't approach the senior staff and say, 'I don't understand'. At that time attitudes were very stiff and hierarchical in all hospitals. However, I think there is probably too much familiarity today.

In the labour room we delivered babies under the supervision of a senior staff midwife or a sister with their hands on top of yours. You never knew what you were doing. However, we were given a wide opportunity to see everything that was difficult and abnormal. If there was something going on that was especially interesting or unusual we were taken to see it.

Miss Betty Burrows was the senior lecturer. She was very well known – a battleaxe! Very clever but stood no nonsense. You were not allowed to be foolish in the slightest. I always think of her sitting at this high desk looking down on the classroom and her hat was right down on her forehead. In Rotten Row they wore strings with a great lacy bow at the side, and that along with their stiff collars made them keep their heads up.

We were taught to deliver the breech in the classroom. We used the phantom pelvis and the phantom fetus and she sat up there during the first part of our lecture, turning the breech because it was extended, and she did all the twisting and turning and getting the legs down, pulling the cord down and so on. I got it so far and I had the doll hanging by the neck. I pulled the cord down and then I thought, 'Now what did she say?' I was standing there pondering and she didn't appear to be paying any attention and never lifted her head, yet she went, 'Go back to your seat instead'. Every breech I have delivered since then, I have remembered. She still haunts me.

I enjoyed the second six months. Things began to fit into place and we weren't so apprehensive. We went out on district for three months. At first we went out with trained staff and then they allowed us to sit with mothers in some very poor homes. We didn't deliver the baby ourselves at that point. We stayed with the mother in labour and assessed the situation. We had little forms with questions and answers and we phoned back to the senior midwife on district and reported what was going on. In those days we were not allowed to do vaginal examinations. We did rectal examinations to assess the dilatation of the os and developed such sensitive fingers that when we had enough practice, when the head was descending we could feel sutures through the rectal wall. When measuring dilatation we used 'fingers' and they use centimetres now. If you measured that the os had dilated, say, four finger breadths, you had to remember a doctor would have bigger hands and his measurements would be different. I can see why they changed to centimetres. Once you reached four fingers, you sent a message saying,'four fingers plus', someone would come out and by then the labour was usually progressing quite well. We had to phone up regularly. There was a lot of poverty in Glasgow and they gave us money to give to the husband to phone. He took the little form which we filled out and phoned the hospital. Sister would ask a question and he would answer what I had written down and this told them it was time to go and join the student. One time a husband was sent with a quick message to say that his wife was 'fully dilated' and he told sister that his wife was 'fully delighted'. Usually a staff midwife came with a medical student as they were in training too and you had a 'case' between you. If one delivered the baby, the other one usually delivered the afterbirth. Then we changed round next time.

Rotten Row had their own caseload within the city boundaries. The other midwives in Glasgow were the Corporation

Midwives. They wore green uniforms and were known as 'Green Ladies'. Rotten Row had a different uniform, their own caseload, usually many more abnormal cases, and used their own senior midwives outside. The Corporation midwives were employed by the Health Board but they trained and supervised midwives from other hospitals like the Western and Rutherglen. Rotten Row pupil midwives went with their own senior staff. But if necessary, we could go with the Green Ladies to make up our numbers. Someone at Rotten Row would phone up and say they had a pupil midwife requiring extra cases. Have you anything to take her to? And then *they* would call in and say, 'I have a case, would you like to send one of your students out?'

At night if we had a call, we went by taxi and met up with the Green Lady if it was her case. I had two emergency deliveries because she didn't get there in time. I felt very important. I was terrified but I don't think the mother noticed. There wasn't time to think about anything except getting on with it. It was a poverty-stricken home. They had called far too late but her mother was there doing her stuff. When I arrived she treated me like the most qualified midwife in the world. I didn't like to tell her I was just a student, so I kept going and she kept patting me on the back and saying, 'Aw, you're a grand girl', and I was just dying a death. It was all very straightforward and easy. It wasn't her first and when the Green Lady came I was just waiting on the afterbirth. I had that twice – both in London Road in Glasgow. It used to be a very busy road for us.

The second time, the taxi dropped me off and the husband came down. They sent you out with the delivery case, the gas and air case and the stitching case. I had all these things to carry and the blue cylinders as well – one under each arm. The husband said, 'Come quick', and he shoved me up all these stairs right to the top. He never even took a case for me, and I'm going up there buckling at the knees. When I got there the baby's head was showing. You just have to get on with it. When the baby was born, the granny wanted to put the baby to the breast. The mother said, 'Ah'm no goin tae feed it, Ah tell ye, Ah'm no goin tae feed it', and the granny turned to me and she said, 'No wonder her weans are wild now. They've been fed on aw that coo's milk and it's no guid for them'.

I enjoyed the district in Glasgow – a very interesting time. I think we had to deliver ten in the hospital in the beginning and twenty out. We had no problem getting cases. There was a lot of poverty. Glasgow was very overgrown by then and Gorbals were still very much there. It seems incredible that we delivered first babies in these wee single-end tenements with bed recesses in the wall in the living rooms and probably one bedroom for the children, the sink with the geyser in the corner, a coal fire, and that was considered acceptable. It wasn't so very long ago.

The proportion of homebirths to hospital was about fifty-fifty. If they had a bed at all and warmth, not central heating then, and some form of hot running water like the geyser in the corner, it was considered OK. If problems showed up during prenatal care they were admitted and then booked for Rotten Row as were older mothers, grande multiparous mothers and medical problems. However if they appeared normal and healthy, they were expected to deliver at home unless they really had nothing.

We had tokens for our fares to go out in the morning in the tramcars and the underground service and do postnatal visits. We also had money for the telephone and we took money with us for gas and electricity meters because sometimes the people didn't have any. Sometimes we had to phone Rotten Row and say, 'Can you bring money? I need to collect the baby's clothes from the pawnshop'. They pawned the clothes hoping to get them back next week. Or, you'd phone to Rotten Row and say, 'Bring clothes. We're short of clothes'. When you visited, things would be all right one week and not the next.

We saw the mother antenatally, but apart from visiting them at home to assess the situation and their needs, mostly they came to the hospital clinics – up Montrose Street outside Rotten Row. It's so steep we used to call it 'induction brae'.

Mothers would be seen by the district midwife, student midwife and doctors once a month till 32 weeks, then once a fortnight and then weekly from 36 weeks. I don't remember much GP input at all.

Life as a midwife

When I qualified I worked as a midwife for two years at the Vert Memorial Hospital – a GP unit – outside Haddington. That was very good and I enjoyed my time there. They had no doctors within the hospital but there were about thirty GP s in East Lothian. Some of them were very old and had been there for quite a long time and some were quite young with new ideas.

Anything complicated was taken into Edinburgh to the Simpson or the Eastern. We mainly did normal midwifery with an occasional breech delivery or low forceps – no ventouse then – and we called the GP if necessary. The GPs did more midwifery then than they do now. They don't seem to be very keen now.

When I first went to the Vert from Rotten Row I was very keen to do everything by the book, proper setting up of trolleys and sterile drapes. I called in an old GP from Dunbar because somebody was requiring some help – just a low forceps delivery. I told him the forewaters were bulging and would probably require rupturing. I set up a trolley and brought it in with all the things required and he looked at it and said, 'What do we need all that for?' I said I thought we'd need it to rupture the membranes. 'Och no.' He scrubbed his hands and just got in there and burst it with his nail. That was my introduction to the old GP-style technique. There were no problems – the baby was fine. Of course midwives ruptured membranes too when necessary, but not like that.

Another time, I was on night duty looking after a prim. She was doing fine and I called in the GP from Gullane – he was a delight – an absolute gentleman, spoke so very precisely and very perjink. He had delivered this girl and her mother before her and he was patting her and saying, 'Now Jennifer you mustn't worry, everything is going to be fine'. He took her pulse – ticking over nicely – and listened in to the fetal heart with the trumpet: 'Yes everything is fine but you need a little bit of help I think'. Then he said, 'Yes, I think we'll have to apply the forks.' I was thinking, 'Forks? What's he talking about?' I'd never heard this term before. I said, 'Excuse me, I have your instruments ready'. In those days everything was boiled and I had them boiled up ready to set my trolley as usual, and he said, 'Oh, I like my own'. I said, 'Right, well, if you give me them I'll boil them'. He took them out and handed them over and I thought, 'Well they're past their best'. I got them scrubbed, and boiled them up. In the meantime the lassie is getting on and he phoned his son-in-law who was going to give the anaesthetic. We had a Boyle's machine but we didn't have a resident anaesthetist and I thought, 'There's no way that he's going to give an anaesthetic surely', but I was mistaken. He said, 'Sister (he called everybody sister), could you get me some castor oil?' I thought, 'This is very strange'. I went away and I came back with a Winchester under my arm. He got a pipette and dropped two drops into her eyes to protect them. Then it dawned on me: 'Oh my goodness he's going to use open mask chloroform'. This was in the late fifties and we didn't see this sort of practice often. The son-in-law, probably a man of around fifty whom I hadn't met before, arrived. He went into the drawer of the Boyle's machine and brought out the open mask. He put the lint over it and got the chloroform and dripped it in. Then he said, 'Now Jennifer we're just going to put you to sleep for a little while'.

The bed we had was one with stirrups and I was all ready to get her legs into stirrups when: 'Not at all sister, I have my own technique'. By this time I was very worried because there was no relief at night, just auxiliaries and one midwife. We got her on to her side and this other fellow gave the anaesthetic. I had to hold her leg. The man with the anaesthetic was up at the top and the old doctor was down at the bottom of the bed practising how he was going to put on these forceps – left over right – and I was now panicking. I wondered, is he going to do an episiotomy? But no, he put the blades in and he started at that side of the bed and he did a manoeuvre and virtually walked all the way round the bottom of the bed and we all ended up on one side of the bed. I was still holding the girl's leg, he's still doing the anaesthetic, and doctor's elbow was in my face. We got a beautiful baby, absolutely perfect, not a mark on it, crying right away, no tear, and a girl who woke up quite quickly from this bizarre anaesthetic and her eyes weren't hurting.

That must have been practice of away back. Probably they did that sort of thing at home years ago. That was the first time I've seen a forceps delivery done like that and afterwards he was so happy for her and she was so delighted with him and said, 'My Mum said you would look after me, Dr K. and I'm so pleased'. He was patting her and saying, 'There there'. Every day he visited twice a day for the first few days, just to take her pulse and hold her hand and say, 'Well done'. He was gorgeous.

The next morning I wrote the report. The Matron was very jittery. She always struck me as being very old although she probably wasn't. She wore a huge veiled cap, very pale-faced and always looked as though she wanted to die. I was giving her the report in the morning and I said to her, 'And last but not least we had Mrs. So-and-So delivered, low forceps by Dr. K.' She went, 'Oh Noooo'. I looked at her and she said, 'Was he all right?' 'Yes,' I said, 'He did very well.' 'Och, she said, 'I wish that man would stop his nonsense.' So she obviously knew but nobody told me that they had these old-fashioned practices. Anyway happy ending. I wouldn't like to see that again but on the other hand, I'm glad I did.

If a GP wanted to be called when someone was going to deliver, we did so. They didn't always want this. We would let them know the situation and how far on in labour the mother was. The doctor usually said, 'Well, if everything is going according to plan, just cope and call me if you need me'. That happened frequently. Often, for first babies they liked to come and they got paid for it too.

Work at the Vert was good experience of the normal side of life. Anything that was too abnormal was sent to Edinburgh and we went in the ambulance with them. All being well, we had the mothers for the ten day postnatal period. With a first baby it was sometimes fourteen. They were in bed for five days and we swabbed them by douching them with Dettol water. We used to have a big trolley with jugs of Dettol douche water and pans underneath it. You put the mother on the bedpan, and you had the douche and swabbing equipment, turned her on her side and examined their stitches and made sure they were healing well.

Homebirths

One of the joys I had of delivering babies at home was this lovely feeling of warmth and a great atmosphere. It was a great joy once we had got the baby and I used to wrap it up all nice and cosy and give everybody a wee quick look. I'd have lovely warm sheets and a warm nightie and bath towels just ready – things for the mother and things for the baby. After everyone had seen the baby I put some oil on it to get the vernix off and I wrapped it up in warm towels and left it there resting. Then I would bed-bath the mother, give her her tooth mug, into her clean sheets and warm nightie, offer her her cosmetic bag, get the hair brushed. Then I would say to usually the Grannie, 'I think your daughter would just love a cup of tea'. While she got that I would bath the baby, dress him in nice warm things, put him in a warm cot and then they could come in.

I would go away on my own to give them time together and do all the cleaning, the slungeing and tidying up and assessing the afterbirth. When I left the house there wouldn't be a speck of blood anywhere. I had a lot of lovely home confinements. Any difficulties that I had I would know when to call a doctor but I think I've been lucky. I always felt reasonably well skilled at the job I was doing.

Callander

I thoroughly enjoyed my job as a nurse/midwife in Callander and the Trossachs. However, when I came, the home delivery levels had dropped and midwifery felt different. People were so full of fear of litigation that it made you stand back from it and that took joy away from the things I had enjoyed in the past. I suppose we didn't stop to worry too much – we just got on with it and did as good a job as you could. Midwifery was meant to be normal until it was proved to be abnormal. Now, it's abnormal until it is proved normal. I feel very sad for midwives and doctors and nurses nowadays. One of the big changes from normal midwifery was the start of almost routine induction of labour and women knew that they were going to be put into labour. That for me was the beginning of abnormality and midwives were included. In those days very very few mothers held their ground.

One who did was a lady who shouldn't have stuck her heels in at all. Whatever I said, she wanted a homebirth but she had everything that recommended a hospital birth. She was red-haired, pale face, first baby, evidence of placenta praevia, and decided to stay at home. My hair was standing on end. Her GP said, 'I'm not having anything to do with this'. But a midwife can't say that. That was a very nasty experience. They talk about stress at work. I remember going to bed thinking, 'Please God, don't phone, I don't want this'. I couldn't sleep worrying about her. I saw her, and trying not to be cross, I said, 'This really isn't fair. You have been given all the advice from everyone. Without painting the picture too black, there is risk'. She said, 'I accept that but I'd rather have the baby born in my house'. I said, 'Yes, I can understand what you're saying but .' In the end we said, 'Will you go to hospital and we will come with you as a compromise?' So we eventually talked her into going into hospital with the midwife, and if everything was fine and normal we would take her home with us.

She phoned at about five o'clock to say she was in labour, and I went out to meet her at the house and she was out walking the dog. By this time my imagination had blood trickling down her legs and all the emergencies in the book. However, she came back home and packed her bag and we went in and I stayed with her for ages. Nothing very exciting happened. She wouldn't have any blood taken to begin with but she eventually did so that we could cross-match it just in case.

When I saw the modern labour room it was very different from what I had been used to. When sister came in she pointed out this machine and that, the oxygen, the thing for checking the bilirubin, blood gases and all. My eyes were like organ stops and I said, 'I don't know how to work the bed pan machine let alone all this. There's no way you're leaving me with that lot. However, put me on top of Ben Ledi with somebody having twins and I would be able to cope'. That was in the late eighties.

Mothers nowadays don't, or won't, rest enough. They possibly think they don't need to. But they get very tired and I think this is why postnatal depression is more now than it was before even though mothers of years ago had so much less.

The input that we gave alongside the GP was much more then. It was a lot of work but worth it. Women's psychological feelings change from week to week and many told you if they were unhappy, or had a problem with their husbands, and didn't know who to turn to. It was worth it to take time and listen to the mother and see how she really was. We used to do visits alternately at home and at the GP's every week or two. We worked very well alongside the GPs – very much a team, working together at the clinics, both palpating and comparing our findings.

Maybe I had the best of it – I think I did. I thoroughly enjoyed all that I did. I've got lots of happy memories – some sad as well but I'm still in touch with lots of babies and mums of years ago. My name was Gordon before I was married and there are so many boys called Gordon round about.

15

'I'M GLAD I CAME BACK'

The midwife whose story this is, was so unhappy with her training as a midwife in 1976 and the treatment of mothers at the time, that she left midwifery and very nearly never returned. Fortunately for midwifery, she did come back. Since then, she has been able to exert her influence along with other midwives to improve the care of mothers, babies and their families in Scotland. She has asked to remain anonymous.

I vowed at the end of my midwifery training that I would never practise as a midwife. I had a horrendous year as a pupil midwife and it took me nine years to come back to midwifery. I went with great expectations, having had a wonderful general nurse training, to a hospital with wartime buildings, and a Victorian nurses' home with attitudes to match. The midwifery tutors were excellent but not able to counteract some of the things that went on on a practical basis.

I started in 1976 and was sent first to the nursery. There was the well-baby nursery and the Special Care nursery downstairs. As a student nurse, although I had done some paediatrics, I had no contact with babies who were ill, in incubators, who needed drips or who needed to be tube-fed. Now, I was alone on duty with the ill babies in a room, sealed off from the main hospital corridor by double doors. This neonatal unit was new, with modern incubators as they had just got rid of the old straw-boxes. Before going in you had to gown-up and put plastic covers on your shoes. Round the wall, there were about eight incubators containing babies, some premature, some with other illnesses. There was no midwife there and I was completely overawed by the situation, absolutely terrified.

'I'm Glad I Came Back'

I lifted the telephone to ask for help. A nursing officer in her late fifties came to the window, opened it and asked what I wanted. I said, 'I'm new, I'm not sure what I'm doing and I would like some help please'. She told me to 'Get on with it' and that was all the help I got.

I had to pass tubes on babies that were tiny. One baby was the size of my hand. I had to give drips to babies. An alarm went in an incubator behind me but I couldn't leave the baby I was dealing with. Because the incubators were ranged round the wall you couldn't observe the other babies in the unit.

Upstairs in the main nursery there were about thirty babies. They all had to be fed, washed , changed and put back in their cots in rotation. Breastfeeding was not in vogue in that hospital. One of the formula milk companies had just brought out a milk which was quoted as 'The next best thing to breast milk' which the hospital had bought, lock, stock and barrel. This was fed to every baby in the well-nursery with no choice given to the mother who only got a quick peek at their babies at visiting time. All the babies went into the well-baby nursery while that mum was in hospital. She never had her baby with her at night and no opportunity to breastfeed unless she fought the system.

There was one Chinese girl who fought the system. Her family, including her other children, visited her and brought her meals in. She breastfed her baby but never received any help because she was not conforming and nobody spoke to her. She was one of the few coloured people in that area and life was made very difficult for her.

In the main, babies stayed in the nursery. Babies were bathed by midwives in the morning in the porcelain sink attached to the wall. Then we all sat with the bottles in a basin of warm water to heat them up and all the babies were bottlefed. Mothers didn't get to feed their babies.

The exception was deformed babies who were allowed to die. They were put into single rooms and fed water until they died. It was horrendous emotionally for me as a human being never mind a student midwife. I don't remember seeing any mums being allowed to be with these babies. I don't remember what happened when the babies died. I think we students were shielded from this but the practice of isolating these babies meant that they had less care than any of the other babies and less chance to be treated as normal human beings. At this time scans were not the norm and one baby had a major spina bifida. It was put in an ambulance and taken up to Glasgow and brought back in the same ambulance before being put into isolation. This baby was only put in the ambulance because the parents had demanded that something be done. Perhaps nothing could have been done for that baby but I remember nursing that baby and nobody coming near.

The unit was a mixture of four-bedded, six-bedded, single and double rooms, divided into antenatal ward, first-stage labour ward and postnatal ward. Women who had not given birth before their due date had to come in and have artificial rupture of membranes (ARM) and syntocinon on that day. When I was part of the antenatal ward staff I worked with these women. They went to the labour ward for induction which was always by ARM. Nobody ever got a medical induction – the oil, bath and enema. Women queued to go into a labour room to have their legs put up in stirrups, to have ARM done. Some women screamed because if the cervix is not ready and is posterior, then they have to howk for it. They were having an invasion of their body for ARM and it did not matter how unready the cervix was.

After this they were taken back to their four-bedded rooms and immediately attached to a syntocinon drip which was turned up regularly with minimal pain relief. Midwives caring for them did fifteen-minute observations on them. We were continually going round doing observations on eight to ten women every day, and when we reached the end we started again. They could have, if you had time, a hot pack on their back or front. Again, if you had time or if their partner or somebody was there – I do remember some partners being there – they could have their back rubbed. They were all on their beds and not allowed up. You could have all these women lying there, either crying quietly, or moaning and groaning. You didn't have time to do the caring that is part of midwifery. That labour suite had four single rooms and one double delivery room, and by two in the afternoon we were delivering without even gloves on because the babies were popping out all over the place without enough staff to cope. We were not allowed to take the women to the labour room until they were in the second stage of labour which meant that they got minimal pain relief, and when they wanted to push you had to say, 'Don't push! Get off the bed and on to the trolley'. We phoned the labour ward to make sure there was a bed. Then, once on the trolley, we pushed them through three or four sets of double doors to the labour ward before they delivered their baby. Woe betide you if they delivered on the bed or the trolley.

One thing which I had great difficulty coping with to the extent that I blanked it out of my mind until recently, was that we had to do rectal examinations on these women. When they were in the first stage of labour, we were not allowed to do vaginal examinations. If we felt they needed to be examined, we had to do it rectally. What an invasion of privacy.

There was no caring. It was just like a sausage factory. They were short of midwives and great emphasis was put on what the doctor said and what he wanted. The women and what they wanted were not considered. Nobody said they didn't want to be induced. They even did inductions on Christmas Day. I was quite far from my family and I was quite happy to work over Christmas and New Year. As I had enjoyed this as a student nurse, I thought it would be a nice experience there as well. It wasn't. There was no happy Christmas feeling. It was just another day with another ten women to be induced and another ten babies to be delivered either by normal delivery or by Caesarean section.

There were twelve of us in the class and four intakes a year. The labour ward was frightening but then that is so for all student midwives. There were the usual frightening dragons of sisters, who probably appeared worse than they really were. We had no problem getting our allocated number of deliveries. Most of us delivered eighty or ninety babies in the year. However, they weren't all supervised. Even if you felt you needed supervision, there wasn't always somebody there to supervise you. Every woman, whether they needed it or not, had an episiotomy. Even if you were delivering unsupervised, it had to be done. We couldn't say, 'No I'm not going to do it'.

One night a woman came in and I admitted her and looked after her in labour. I was delivering her unsupervised. The head came out and as you do, I looked at it. I thought, there's something funny about this head but I don't know what it is. Then the body was born and it was one of the worst spina bifida babies I have ever seen. I didn't know what to do. Although I was well on in my training and in that area there was a fair number of abnormal babies, I had never delivered one before and I didn't know how to cope.

The mother dealt with the problem. She could see from my face there was something wrong and she said, 'Is everything OK?' I stammered, 'Well, well, I'm not sure'. She touched my arm and said, 'Has it got spina bifida?' and I said, 'Yes.' 'It's all right, hen,' she said, 'I've got one at hame like that. Another yin'll no make ony difference.' I still thank that woman. I wonder how she got on. With two spina bifida babies to look after, her life must have been miserable. But she was able to acknowledge how I felt. I don't know how I got through the rest of the night and I don't honestly remember what happened to that mother. Nowadays probably it wouldn't happen but then, scans were only in their infancy and not for everybody. There were no scanning facilities at the hospital, and even if she had fallen into the criteria of the research project on obstetric ultrasound scanning, we were too far away from the research centre. There was nobody to talk it through with me. Everybody felt there was nothing they could do to change things so why talk about it?

It was such a nightmare that I nearly gave up at the end of three months. Then I thought, 'No, I don't give up that easily. I'll get to the end of this'. It affected my work and the tutorial staff told me my work wasn't up to standard. I was able to say why. I felt this wasn't the way to treat women and I really didn't want any part of it. I felt very awkward about the way women were treated and the things I was expected to do.

The tutors listened but were unable to do anything. However, they did give me a study plan which I worked to. I studied every morning and every night for a set length of time to make sure that I hit the basic required standard and hopefully pass all the exams.

While I was in the postnatal ward we had quite a lot of women who had lost their babies. The high level of abnormality in that area meant a high level of miscarriage. They were not treated well either. Women, having miscarried at home, came in, several of them with their miscarriage in a bag. Before they were examined they had to have a shave, enema and bath whatever else happened.

They were put in a bed and given a D&C if they needed one. They and any other postnatal women who complained of any ailment were prescribed Valium. The doctors' understanding of women and women's emotions appeared minimal and they seemed to think that the fashionable Valium was the panacea for all ills. Everybody was put on Valium, whether they needed it or not, to calm them down, make them sleepy and forget what had happened to them.

They had a ward – a long Nightingale ward in a Nissan hut type of building – away from the main area of the hospital, kept for women who had had miscarriages. They also carried out terminations there. All these women were in the ward together and all physically given the same treatment. However, there were a whole lot of different emotional problems going on in the same area. Nobody bothered about what these women were going through. It was part of our training to be in theatre while terminations were going on and also understand what happened when we were doing a late termination, that is one which was after twelve weeks. We were all involved unless we had very strong religious reasons not to. Most of us felt under duress not to refuse in case we got a black mark which might affect the rest of our training.

Some of the women in the area went to local maternity homes, but since then these have been shut down as in many other areas. They were a mixture of GP homes and those run by midwives. As a student, I never went out to any of these because I couldn't afford a car until about six months into my training. Some of my colleagues who lived locally went to the maternity homes and saw birth from a totally different viewpoint.

I enjoyed my time on community because it was a different way of working. It only lasted about a month – two weeks during the first half of the training and then two weeks towards the end. It was not long but the training at that time was only a year and they had a lot to cram in. My community midwife who covered a rural area with farmers' wives who might have been interested in home births, made it very clear from the start that she was not in favour of them. I never saw her do an early antenatal visit as all antenatal bookings were done by the time that I came in contact with the women. We did some clinic work and home postnatal visits but nothing else. My view of midwifery must have been very skewed.

There was one woman aged nineteen who already had one baby. She was having triplets by another partner. It was around New Year. I had been at a party and came in and was told to go to theatre to be part of the emergency Caesarean section team. The way that woman was treated was appalling. She did have problems with her family, but they had already picked out a foster family for the triplets. However, the social work care had not teamed up with the hospital care. There were big banner headlines in the papers, 'They are taking my babies away from me'. I don't know what happened to these children. Have they spent their lives in a children's home? How is that mother feeling now? Nobody cared or that's the way it appeared.

But perhaps having created a bit of a stink, she got a bit more caring than the girls coming to have their babies adopted. It was a seaside area. Lots of girls came, ostensibly to work for the season, and during that time they would come in and have their babies and leave. They had no help. There was no social work care, no aftercare, nothing. They just came in, did the deed and were away. Some don't want extra care but a lot of girls do. If their baby was going for adoption, the baby was taken out as soon as it was born and kept in the well-baby nursery. It was fed, washed and cared for like all rest until it went away and the mother was never allowed to see it.

The only stillbirth that I remember was one that happened to a girl who had gone to school with me. She married, moved to this area and had a stillborn baby. I was working in the postnatal ward and there she was. I remember treating her kindly but I don't remember anybody else doing so. She was put in a single room and she cried. But then everybody cried. I was told, 'Leave her to cry. She needs to cry. She does her crying in here and then she won't cry when she goes home'. I made a point of going in and talking to her although nobody told me what to say or how to say it but you find the words. Nobody liked what I was doing. I was kept busy so that I would be kept out of the way and she went home in a few days and I never saw her again for a long while. She was treated just as other girls were treated. There was not enough staff and no time, to care. There was a real feeling of, 'Brush it under the carpet, forget it happened and you're young enough, you can have another one'.

At this time there were lots of women's groups evolving like the National Childbirth Trust. Empowerment of women was happening – books were talking about women and feminism, and even though I'm not a 'feminist' there's a happy medium. Women when they're pregnant, when they're in labour and just after, need to be mothered themselves, for their own sakes and in order to help them to mother. They need the caring that goes along with midwifery.

Last year I returned to that hospital on a study day and it's a changed place. It has been renovated and the labour area is dramatically different. Hopefully the practice and the care of the students is also dramatically different as I didn't feel that I was cared for. I don't think this hospital was typical of maternity units in Scotland at the time. My sister trained as a midwife elsewhere in Scotland and when I questioned her about it, what she described was totally different.

The whole experience for me was horrendous. I had a calendar and scored it off night and morning to help me get through the year. When I got my final pass papers in the post I went and blew all the money I had saved on a foreign holiday just to enjoy the experience and the feeling of freedom because it was like having been in prison for a year.

As well as reacting to the way women were treated, I fought against the Victorian attitudes in the nurses' home. In other places you were treated and held responsible as an adult. I had been in charge of my life for several years. Why should I have to sign in and out? Why should I have to justify where I was going or who with? Why should I have to go to the senior matron's office to collect my mail and tell her who it was from? It was not a happy year. I vowed – if that's what they do to women, I want no part of it.

I went back into general nursing and continued into teaching and research which gave me a broader view of nursing and a high-flying career. I was also aware that I had a health problem which meant that I might not be able to have children, and a high-stress career would not help this. So, about to be married, I turned my prospects upside down and looked for a part-time job as a staff midwife. The lady then in charge of this hospital knew my career history and invited me for interview. She said, 'I can't give you a sister's job'. I told her that all I wanted was a part-time job until I had children and she took me on.

Staff midwife, 1983

This hospital was wonderful. I was quite frightened to begin with but I heard what it was like through some of the midwives. I was aware that the staffing levels were different and the way they cared for mothers in labour was different. They didn't shave mothers any more, or do enemas. Women were allowed to move around in labour and partners were welcomed. When I was in training they were only allowed into the first- stage room if they were assertive enough to make their presence felt. To begin with I was amazed at the caring that went on. The formidable old dragons were there but they could show their caring side too.

The number of midwives was astonishing. Antenatal clinics were staffed by up to seven midwives. Midwives delivered the babies and stitched up afterwards if necessary. Midwives helped mothers put babies to the breast. I hadn't really seen much of breastfeeding – just what we had talked about in the classroom. There was still a high proportion of bottlefeeders but now the mothers had the choice and there was more than one type of milk available. The whole way women were looked after was different.

I worked for four days a week until my son was born and then three days a week until my daughter was three. The job I'm in now came up in the late 1980s and I thought long and hard about it. I knew if I didn't take it somebody else would and it really suited my qualifications and experience. By this time family life had changed, my health problems had resolved and I had my children. I applied for the job and went for the interview thinking, 'I'll try it for six months and if I can't cope with it I'll give it back'. Even when they offered me the job I said, 'Yes', and at the back of my mind that thought was there – and I'm still here.

Labour ward here is lovely. Women have a room to themselves for the duration of their labour. Some women, particularly if they have delivered in other areas and are coming here for their second or third baby, think, 'This is where the baby is born but where do I go before then?' We can say to her, 'This will be your room for however long you're here'. They can do what they want and you can talk about the beanbags and different positions for labour, and if they don't want the bed in the room we can take it out.

In my previous hospital I hadn't come across the National Childbirth Trust although I was aware of their existence.

Although I was quite sympathetic because we seemed to be saying the same thing, sometimes I felt the way they were saying it was a bit over the top. In time, the gap has narrowed, things have improved and women can choose and tell us what they want.

Sometimes we suggest things that women and their partners can't cope with, such as skin-to-skin contact, or the partner cutting the cord. Some men can't cope with that yet, but the pendulum has swung the other way. There is still a fair amount of clinical supervision from the consultants because this is still a consultant unit. However, in this unit the midwives have a good say in what goes on. It's a totally different experience working here and I'm awfully glad I came back as a midwife.

16

STUART HISLOP

*Until 1975 midwifery was one of the professions where
discrimination on the grounds of gender was permitted. It
was illegal in Britain for any man to practise midwifery unless
he was a medical practitioner or in an emergency. The Sex
Discrimination Act was passed in 1975 and removed the
barriers to men becoming midwives, although some restric-
tions remained about where they should practise. Two pilot
schemes, each including male pupil midwives, were started in
1977 – one in England and one in Scotland. Stuart Hislop was
the first Scotsman to train in midwifery. He qualified as a
midwife in 1981.*

I have always been fascinated with the process of childbirth. In 1980 Frances and I didn't have children although
we both wanted them. The subject of conception and
birth really interested me and it seemed perfectly natural
to work on a professional basis with people who were
having babies. I never had a problem or any inhibition with
being a male midwife as people always insisted on calling
me.

My background was in nursing. I started in psychiatry,
moving from there to train as a general nurse. I was a staff
nurse for a while before going into midwifery. I knew no
Scotsmen had done midwifery but it seemed right for me to
do it at that time. When the Sex Descrimination Act was
passed in 1975, and then the EEC Directives were passed in
1976, there was an initial interest in the media that males
could now do midwifery. I didn't look on myself as a pioneer,
but being a Scotsman doing midwifery in a Scottish hospital
did attract some attention.

Going into midwifery made me think carefully about gender issues. Usually it's women who are discriminated against. People tend not to think so much about discrimination happening the other way round. From the start the Health Board insisted that we didn't need chaperones. In the London hospital also pioneering male midwifery, we heard they employed people to act as chaperones for the male midwives. A few of the staff here seemed to agree with this, and I took their attitude personally as I didn't like the implication that I couldn't be trusted with a woman in labour.

I was far too busy learning about the mechanics of child-birth, and I found what they were insinuating quite insulting. I was immersed in the job, and as I handled the babies and worked with the mothers I never thought of gender at all. I was the person doing the job. I think the people I was working with felt the same way. This seemed to prove that the person with the skills is important, not his or her gender. We'd never think about it if it were a doctor – we're used to it. It was in all the pamphlets and information packs – Forth Valley employs male student midwives and saying what to do if they had any objections. I was only once refused to do a procedure in the whole time I was in the maternity unit. That was for an enema that a woman needed. I withdrew and somebody else did it.

However, I had no real problem with other members of staff about being a man. One of my colleagues said I changed her view and that you can't make generalisations like 'males can't be good'. Attitudes *were* changing, and by the time I started midwifery there was probably less tension. Possibly the profile of midwifery in general was raised because of the publicity of letting men enter the profession. People spoke about the expertise and skills involved and midwifery got quite a good press – maybe for the wrong reasons. Every now and again the subject would come up again and the men took it turn about to see who was going to have their picture in the papers! This went on during most of the year I was there as a student. It was an eventful year. It was quite cosmopolitan with Australians and a New Zealander and ourselves, and as a group we balanced the demands of the social life and the demands of study and the job as well. I really enjoyed it.

All areas of midwifery seemed to be part of the environment with which I was familiar, except they concentrated on pregnancy and birth. To be part of the business of delivering a baby was a huge buzz. It was good being with a couple in the labour ward and building up a rapport with them. They were interested in me and I was interested in them and at the end of this period if you got to deliver their baby you felt very privileged. I still see children who are 'my deliveries', and people still stop and speak to me. They knew I was doing my job and there were no inhibitions, no feeling that I was intruding on something that I shouldn't have been. I knew my place, worked hard to do the job as well as I could and acquired an ability to be sensitive to the woman's needs at that time.

There appeared to be a geniune fascination with, 'How does a man become a midwife?' People could understand a nurse but they couldn't fathom this. Even after I explained how I came to it, they wanted to talk about it. It was good to have people so interested in what I was doing. But during that year I behaved like any other student and got on with what I was doing. It was very important to me not only to be accepted in college and complete the course but to prove I could do the job as a midwife. Many people just got the qualification and moved on. For me that wouldn't have been enough. I had to prove to my colleagues that I could work with them as an equal and be regarded as a midwife. That's why I stayed and practised as a midwife for about six months before moving into education.

As a midwife I worked on night duty on the postnatal ward. It was a good experience, very rewarding and very demanding. We were very busy. I would sit down at about half-past five or six in the morning, my first chance to write up the notes to hand over to the day staff. There were fewer staff on at night and yet there would be the same amount of work, as there were always admissions from the labour ward.

It was also a good opportunity to talk to mothers in the night. Problems loom large during the night and the psychological care given then was as important as any thing else. One woman burst out crying. I said, 'What's wrong?' She said, 'Look how easily you handle that baby and I'm so clumsy'. I said, 'But you've just had the baby. I've been handling babies for a long time. It takes time to be confident'. I went away and really thought about this. It was good to feel the skills in oneself, but what negative effect did it have on someone else? I became very aware, in my psychological care of mothers, of their unsureness of themselves especially when they were tired and morale was low.

I tried to assess what the women needed, like having their baby in the nursery for a night. I saw them becoming increasingly drained and would offer to look after the baby for them and promise to waken them up if necessary. I felt it was important to discuss this as they could be up at night with the baby for quite long periods. I did the same with the Caesarean section mothers. I never felt that by, say, the third day they should be at any particular stage of recovery. I looked at the person first and assessed them. Communication too is important. I always said, 'Please buzz if you need me', and they did. You got to know the mothers very well especially if they were in for five days and you saw wee patterns emerging. Sleep deprivation seemed to affect the psychological wellbeing of the mother and I liked to take into account the needs of each mother rather than official policy about always rooming in. It was wonderful to see someone after they had had a good night's sleep. You saw a different, really refreshed person. It seemed so important and natural to make sure they got a good night's sleep. Maybe I just don't like being sleep-deprived.

The breastfeeding mothers were making an extra effort but they were so tired. I saw no harm in a baby missing one breast feed and letting the mother get a good night's sleep. Obviously you took the mother's wishes into account. But they needed a lot of support. They were always worried. Breastfeeding is a natural thing but you can't measure a breastfeed.

Stuart Hislop

When it came to helping a mother put her baby to the breast for feeding, I think the word 'professional' is the one to use. When you saw the breast there you were thinking about fixing the baby. It may be unusual for a man to stand and be there but it was perfectly natural and I think I probably did reasonably well. I can't count the number of times I've assisted a mother put her baby on the breast. I would never do anything that was inappropriate. I made a very conscious decision that I must never give off the wrong signals to women and I must never give the impression that there was any other reason for being there, and I would have died a death if I had ever allowed that line to be crossed.

I think the way we were socialised into midwifery is different from male doctors into medicine. Male doctors don't seem to have had the same problem as male midwives. There was always the feeling, 'Oh, you're a doctor, therefore . . .' I don't think they think so deeply about this particular aspect – clinical dimension, yes, but their relations to women patients, no. I remember reading about a female medical student saying if she had her way all junior male doctors would be taken into a room, put in a lithotomy position and have a woman walk in, grab them by the testicles and walk out again without saying a word.

I hope being a midwife helped me empathise more with women. Frances and I didn't have children at the time. One time as a student, I was working in the labour ward and there was a thirteen-week fetus waiting to be taken to the lab. I happened to walk into the room where this fetus was. Frances had had four or five miscarriages, one of them eleven weeks and one fourteen weeks. I stood and looked at this fetus and thought, 'That's what we lost' and I felt very inadequate because I hadn't really thought about what it was like for Frances. Although I had had the lectures and the theoretical knowledge, I hadn't realised what I was maybe trying to come to terms with. That was one of those experiences in life that stays with you, and I felt I understood in a way for the first time what it was like to lose a baby. I don't think many men can appreciate this and I don't tell people this very easily.

Then I realised that I would always be male and maybe anything I do would have to be with a particular sensitivity as I would always have a male reaction. I think I began to understand then what it must be like for a woman, and I realised that males sometimes don't appreciate this, not as a fault or a failing, but as a characteristic. Although I'm still a man, I feel I now see some things a little differently. I think a man can be good enough as a midwife but needs to try and be more empathetic. I was really blown away by that experience because I really thought I had dealt with the miscarriages.

The midwife occupies a very privileged position, far more so than in nursing. Midwifery skills are not just about the mechanics of labour – it's the whole experience of having a baby which we can help to become meaningful. There are still people who come up to me years on and say, 'Remember me?' They always say, 'You were with me'. You occupy a very important place often for a very short space of time.

When I came into midwifery a wind of change was blowing and it was realised that women who came into hospital had rights. I was handed 150 mg. of Pethidine by the sister who had drawn it up and told, 'Go and give it to that person', with no discussion about whether she wanted painkillers or not. Although there was not too much of that, it was there. However, that attitude was being challenged by mothers and midwives. I saw incredible acts of kindness and wonderful role-models. The sister on the ward where I worked as a midwife was kindness personified. She had a wonderful approach and to her, the mothers came first. I got on fine working with her and was allowed to be responsible for those I was looking after. I came across many midwives who were very able, able to teach, who cared about their clients and midwifery practice and had done so all their lives. There were people who you wouldn't want to change because they were good at what they were doing, whether you call it modern or old practice. However, in the seventies routine procedures seemed to dominate and this was being challenged quite aggressively. Some people hated the idea of change. Midwives were beginning to realise that they were enjoying a good press because of good things they were doing. Factory production was going. Midwives were beginning to stand up for mothers and themselves.

Generally speaking we had a good rapport with the medical staff. A couple of junior doctors were absolute pains. The rest of them were charming and worked closely with the midwives, respecting their opinions and recognising that most of the deliveries were in our control. Also, the mother was being brought into things far more. In the past it had been doctors and midwives deciding. Now it was a real partnership between midwives and the mothers. This had been going on for some time and many of the midwives were excellent.

I saw a woman who had been in labour for twenty-eight hours. The consultant was unhappy about it but because the mother had had such a horrendous experience in a maternity unit before, he said, 'OK, we'll let her have her head'. She was exhausted and not everyone agreed. However, she delivered vaginally. She seemed fine after, and although it wasn't a perfect birth, everyone was aware that this was what she wanted. She wasn't on a drip, she didn't want anything associated with the previous time and she delivered the baby herself. She was tired by the end of a very long haul but she remained in control. This highlights a very important thing about being a midwife. That is, you can enable someone to be in control of their labour and birth rather than taking over. Good midwives know the time to *suggest*, rather than tell, and it's not that the person has lost control – but that you were there to help at the right time. It's difficult to decide how you get just that right moment. It's quite a skill, and a challenge.

The fathers were fascinating. They liked being part of this discussion, that they were being included in what was going on. You really got to know about people, what their life was like, their expectations, what they did. I was amazed at the number of people who were unemployed at that time. I had never been unemployed and I learned a lot.

There was a terrible situation I look back on with regret. A woman came in in labour. We couldn't hear the fetal heart, were almost sure that she would have a stillbirth, and the place was really busy. One of the sisters said, 'Could you go and phone up the partner and get him in?' I phoned and I said, 'Hello, my name's Stuart Hislop, I work in the labour ward in Falkirk. Would you come in to be with your wife?' The response was, 'Aye come on Geordie, that's a good wind-up'. I had this sinking feeling. I said, 'Look, I do understand that people play practical jokes. If you have a problem I'll put the phone down and you phone back to the labour ward in Falkirk', and I gave him the number. I eventually managed to convince him that he was really needed here. All the time I knew that his baby was dead and he thought he was getting his leg pulled. The cruelty of that situation really got to me. I thought, 'That wouldn't have happened if it had been a female doing the phoning'. My immediate guilt was because I was a male midwife and I was in the wrong place at the wrong time. Then I thought, 'Nonsense, it could have been a doctor or anybody making that phone call'. But I took days to get over that. All I could think was this poor guy who thought he was getting his leg pulled.

Most of the time everything was great. One night I sat with a guy for two and a half hours in Stirling. He was drunk and sister didn't want to phone the police. The woman insisted he wasn't getting to see her. The guy was drunk although not aggressive, but if we had phoned the police he would have been arrested. We sat together for a good while and I gave him a cup of tea. Eventually we felt he was sober enough to get him off the premises. So we said, 'We'll get you a taxi, get you home. Come back tomorrow. Maybe things will be better in the morning'. Sister genuinely didn't want him to be arrested, especially when he wasn't aggressive-drunk. He was sad-drunk, daft-drunk. But if he had gone upstairs he might have made a nuisance of himself and we couldn't take that chance. I felt sorry for him. This poor guy had had a bit of a row, got himself very drunk, thought he was going to put it right that night and would probably have made things worse. We stopped him from being arrested but equally we felt it was our duty not to let him go in. It was a difficult situation.

No matter how robust or able you are, childbirth takes its toll. This was brought home to me one day when I went in to see someone who I knew was a GP. She'd had her baby a few days before and she was crying. She's a very able, capable person. I said to her, 'Are you all right? Is there anything I can do?' She said, 'I'm just having one of these moments'. That was all she needed to say. As I walked away I thought if someone as able as she is can feel like that, it doesn't matter how strong you are, childbirth has a terrific effect on you. People need help. It's very hard work having a baby and the midwife is dealing with someone who very often isn't feeling excited and happy . They feel as though their self-esteem is in their boots, and often feel very inadequate. To be with them in this situation is an incredible privilege and it is so easily open to abuse. For a midwife to be able to help is critical. I meet with most of the current midwifery groups here at Stirling University and try hard to get some of these thoughts on psychological care over to them.

Bringing men into midwifery fitted into the changes that were happening at the time, the questioning, challenging and raising of awareness of what was going on in the childbirth arena. People were beginning to ask, 'Is it really appropriate in the first place?' It was all part of the change and growth of the time.

Being a man in midwifery, I was given a lot of attention and feedback. It was very positive and could have become quite addictive. However, I would hope never to get carried away with this as I realised there was more to it than the sideshow. The most important thing for me was what I was doing. To this day I'm very proud of what I did during those eighteen months and it's a nice part of my life to look back on.

17

ELIZABETH CARSON

Elizabeth Carson trained as a midwife in Glasgow and practised as a midwife in two hospitals in Glasgow before going to live and work in Oban. This turned out to be a very different way of life and midwifery practice.

I did my training in Glasgow and completed in 1961. I practised as a midwife first in Belvidere Hospital, a GP unit, and then in Stobhill. In 1981 we moved to Oban and I got a post at the local maternity unit soon after. At that time it was a six-bedded self-contained GP Unit in a large granite house originally owned by a local baker who made his money from the diamond mines in South Africa and gifted to the Health Board by the family about forty-five years ago.

The house was beautiful with fabulous views over the bay and lovely marble fireplaces of different colours in all twelve rooms. At night we didn't shut the curtains so that the patients could lie in bed and watch the sunset over Mull. The maternity unit was there until five years ago when we moved to the new hospital in Oban. The GPs were in close contact with one coming daily for morning coffee after surgery and to visit her patients. Another came to visit his patients earlier, before I went off night shift in the morning. Now, as it is a midwife-led unit, we still have GP cover but if we require a GP we phone and let them know. We have about sixty-five to seventy deliveries per year and a few years ago we got to an exceptional eighty-four. Unfortunately, a couple of years ago, due to finances, the GPs were no longer willing to cover the patients from outlying areas. Some mothers therefore had to be transferred and delivered in Glasgow or wherever they chose. We lost quite a few deliveries then.

Elizabeth Carson

Last October (1999) we got the service back because Dr Wilson, wife of one of our local GPs, and an absolute gem, agreed to take on medical cover for these patients. They're midwife-cared-for unless there is an emergency. We can phone Dr Wilson up with a problem and she will come out day or night.

We have twelve midwives on the staff, some part-time, and approximately 200-250 women on our caseload at one time. We deal with normal midwifery except for a few exceptions when an emergency occurs too late for the mother to be moved.

It's eighty miles to our consultant unit at the Vale of Leven Hospital and a hundred miles to the Queen Mother's Hospital in Glasgow. If a mother goes to either of these units, she's usually away until she has delivered and then generally returns within forty-eight hours. Occasionally someone will come back within twenty-four hours even after a section, quite shellshocked because of the journeys. The patients are so delighted to be back, they don't care. It's wonderful for us as we can carry on with the postnatal care.

We had forty-five deliveries in 1998. Last year (1999) we went up to fifty-two because we have our outlying patients back. The more we keep up the productivity, the happier the powers that be are with the service. GP units are quite costly although we're constantly watching and economise where we can.

When I started here they had double-duty and triple-duty nurses/midwives covering the outlying areas. Now the midwives based in the unit work in the community as well. Recently we started midwife clinics in hospital which have been very popular. The uptake by the mothers has been so successful that next year we're hoping to have an extra day. It's run every week on a Thursday between 11a.m. and 7p.m. so that women who are working can come. The extra day will possibly be a Saturday to help people from outlying areas in the town doing their shopping. We cut back on the community service where we can, and think we can justify this extra improved service for the community. In a recent study regarding what patients wanted, the staff found they were keen to have a midwife visit them at home. So a midwife visits a couple of times in a pregnancy. You learn much more about a mother and her circumstances at home than in the clinic.

Sometimes quite a lot of the day is spent on the road because midwives cover a wide area as far as Dalmally, as far down as Clachan-Seil to Cuan Ferry, Easdale, Kilmelford and Ardfern. Distance curtails the number of visits a midwife can do in a day, especially at the height of the tourist season or if it's bad weather.

Within the department we try and have two midwives per delivery. During the day, if the community midwife is out she can be called back to be the second midwife at a delivery. I have worked for the last number of years as night sister and now, am by myself with a midwife on call. When I need her I call her out and she will come to do the delivery with me before going home. I try not to call her out for too long. That backfired two weeks ago when a girl who was 7-8 centimetres, second baby, came in after being in labour most of the day. I called the second midwife at twenty past eleven and baby was born at ten past five the following morning. By that time the second midwife had been on the go about twenty-four hours. I felt bad about it but there was nothing you could do. The mother just took her time delivering.

Two years ago because of cost, the night-auxiliary was taken to Care of the Elderly and there is an auxiliary rostered there available for us if necessary. On my own, I have a maximum of five – two mothers and three babies. If, for any reason, I feel that I'm not coping with that, I can ask for her to come.

We have a very happy working unit here and know each other well. We started team midwifery about ten years ago and have worked like that since then. The patients think it's great and talk about us being a first-class hotel. If we're full, which is six mothers and six babies, the one midwife would usually have auxiliary cover during the day.

Five years ago the new hospital in Oban was opened up and our small unit of six beds moved from the beautiful house to within the hospital. What we gained out of the move was the theatre round the corner. Although they did some forceps deliveries in the old maternity unit, in most emergencies where anything operative was required, the patient was transferred across the town to the hospital. We had the odd emergency when somebody came in bleeding and we sadly lost two babies one after the other some years ago. That was very traumatic for everybody. Apart from losing her baby, one of the mothers nearly lost her life. Being eighty miles from a consultant unit, you can't shift certain patients out. We now have a theatre round the corner which is wonderful. It's the only gain that we got out of being in a big new modern hospital. That, and a beautiful new incubator. It means we can do the sections, forceps and twin deliveries which happen occasionally in the theatre there. In an emergency, if the roads are closed and you can't get out of the town, or if the helicopter can't fly because of the wind conditions, you have to get on with it. After each situation like that we have a discussion with the GPs to see what else could be done to change or improve things.

The Health Board looks at the financial implications of the maternity service every so often and examines what we're providing in relation to cost. They won't close it but they may reduce it. If they contracted the service too much, the women who know what they can choose when it comes to having babies might refuse to go elsewhere. The huge distance involved to the consultant units would be very unpopular with patients who require normal midwifery. Then there might be other problems for the staff, like unplanned home deliveries, or emergency situations where the women might leave it too late and not want to travel further. Some patients must have consultant care and therefore must go to a consultant unit. Which one, will depend on what the Health Board decide. However, because of the rural area you can't do away with the service totally and they will need to keep some sort of service going in Oban . . .

One of the suggestions is that all prims will go to a consultant unit. However, we have one or two who decide every year that although this is their first baby, they're not leaving their community. They're told that if they need to go to a consultant unit for any reason, they should heed the advice. It only happens occasionally. The labour slows down, we are not allowed to use syntocinon and the policy at the moment is that the patient should be transferred.

We are fortunate that in the last five years we have only had one delivery en route. It happened in the car park in Tarbert. The mother had been with us for over twenty-four hours and her labour slowed and stopped. We transferred her out and she got sixty miles, as far as Tarbert. It wasn't all that far from the Vale of Leven and they went there for mother and baby to be checked. That doesn't happen often now. It used to happen before because the journey took longer on the bad roads. It can be quite a difficult decision to make as every labour is different. We have had the odd situation when about thirty miles down the road we've turned round and come back. Rather than deliver in the ambulance she's better delivering in the unit.

I think mothers are having their babies more quickly now than forty years ago, possibly because they're healthier and fitter. They're certainly better informed now and that helps. We use very little in the way of analgesia for our patients. Even prims often only have Entonox. When I started, prims were sedated with whatever was the regime of the day. I think in the past they listened to stories from their grandmothers and mothers. Now the mothers are better informed from reading, television and other media and their midwives. Some of them are very keen to do anything that will give them a better labour. They understand the process better, and understanding gives confidence, all helped by antenatal tests and scans. Also, you hear them talking about 'midwives' now. The whole profile of birth, maternity care and midwifery is much higher than before.

We have very few home deliveries, probably because the mothers like the unit so much. We had one last year (1999), a second baby and all went very well. Home deliveries are quite costly. We have to have an extra midwife on call and that puts our budget up dramatically. We wouldn't deny anybody a homebirth but it could affect the whole community. If it costs more, then the Health Board might have to reduce the service. An alternative option could be, come in and have your baby and go home in six hours. We try and make the unit like a home from home and the mothers in labour are up and about and very free. They might have to sit still for a wee while for a CTG tracing, but other than that they're not confined to bed, they're up parading about, watching telly, reading magazines, having a cuppa, their husband or granny or a friend is with them and sometimes more than one.

Last year we acquired a birthing pool. A group of mostly NCT clients decided they wanted to do something about this. Before that, mothers wanting a waterbirth hired their own pool which they brought into the hospital. Some of the GPs were not so keen but some of the midwives are quite keen, and so is our manager Betty MacIntyre who runs this service. The birthing group, called 'Pool Together', collected money through raffles and other means, and the Health Board organised the installation of a proper plumbed-in pool. We had two waterbirths last year and one booked shortly and we have our own protocol written out about the mother being in the water. Our manager oversees it with whatever midwife is on duty. For some it doesn't work – the mother might be past her dates or have other complications. However, some of the patients are very satisfied with the pool and feel they got what they wanted.

We try to give women all the options, advice and guidance and they choose for themselves what they would prefer. Some need to be pointed in the right direction. For instance, if you have a baby who needs specialised care, we don't have a paediatrician. Our GPs will come out willingly and do their best for their patient but you have to look at all points of view. Nowadays, people plan their families quite carefully. Then sometimes they don't listen to advice. However, on the whole we have very few hiccups. It's wonderful.

Before I came to Oban I worked in Stobhill in the days of induction. We did four inductions per day every day in the

1970s and 1980s. Inductions were 'progress'. With retrospect that was not progress. Patients with one or two children were having induced and accelerated labour and they told us afterwards that this was more traumatic than having their first baby, born with no problems. They found induction quite devastating. But that was what happened at the time. We were in a consultant unit, there were six consultants, everything was on tap, with paediatrician, anaesthetist, blood services and labs all there.

In Oban they were not on tap. I hope I became a better midwife when I came to Oban because of this although it was quite a culture shock. If I wanted a lab, I called somebody out. We didn't have an anaesthetist. We have one now. We still don't have a paediatrician. If you had a problem with a baby, you called out a GP or the midwives on duty coped. We have to think differently and anticipate. We give whole care, antenatally, intrapartum and postpartum, rather than specialising. I like the way we work in Oban very much. I have been back to a couple of consultant units for refresher courses and found it very high-tech, very pushed and short-staffed. That's probably the way I worked before and didn't realise it at the time.

When I started my training, antenatal care was not as it is now with scans. We were presented with things then like undiagnosed twins, placenta praevia. Now, we can predict when a woman is going to have a ten-and-a-half-pound baby and can decide what we're going to do for her. So, as you can plan better, the care is better. By the time I reached Oban, antenatal care had improved. We have a scan machine which the consultant uses when he comes to the clinic and are getting a new one. Some of the midwives and GPs can scan too. It's good for the mothers to come and have their scan here where they have a kent face.

In Oban we have to provide emergency maternity cover for a large area of Argyll and the islands. We can have lifeboat, helicopter and ambulance escort. Ambulance escorts are usually the norm and in an emergency a midwife would go too. To be moved in an emergency can be very traumatic for a mother and her family. Also, a midwife escorting the mother in the ambulance has to be away from the unit for five-and-a-half or six hours.

If a mother is able and if she's booked elsewhere, a couple might go on their own in their own transport. A lot of them do this nowadays, especially in early labour. We make sure they know where they can get help and I usually check that they know what road they are going and where phone boxes are. If they do run into difficulties, they have somewhere to go. It's a long road. Up to half way I tell them to phone us if there's a problem, and after that I tell them to phone in to their destination. They could be going to a consultant unit in Edinburgh, or Raigmore, which rarely happens. It's usually to the Vale of Leven or Glasgow – eighty or a hundred miles – because that's where they're booked. We had someone going to the Queen Mother's in Glasgow and they had to call into the Vale because they didn't get that far. We've had patients going to Edinburgh and they've had to call into Stirling for the same reason. I check that they know what they're doing. If the driver isn't happy with it, then we get an ambulance to take them. They could be on holiday. If they've gone into labour on holiday it depends how far on they are and how far away from home they are. We wouldn't turn them away.

Some choose to go back to their family to have the baby. So they go back home to Raigmore, Edinburgh or Glasgow and they may choose to go in labour. That gets discussed during their antenatal care but it's their choice. They may not want to go before labour and sit and wait, which used to happen. When Stobhill was open, mothers used to go and sit in Stobhill for a week or two before they delivered. So, people from here, booked elsewhere, go in labour and an ambulance is not the best place for a labouring patient. There was a time when the midwife sat on a stool in the middle of the ambulance and attended to her patient. Since the Skye accident everybody has to be belted in. If you need to attend to your patient, you get the ambulance to stop before you do so. Anyway, what are you going to do if you find a problem? You're not going to be able to do anything at the top of the

Rest and be Thankful, other than notify your intended destination that you have a problem and to be ready for you.

When we use the lifeboat, a GP usually goes out with a midwife and a small incubator. Until fairly recently it was considered just part of the job. As a result of the Skye accident we're all taking a close look at what we were doing. We have had talks with Health and Safety officers and now we're having training. So I've now been out on a lifeboat, which I hadn't done in all the time I've been here as a midwife. Five months ago I went out in a brand-new, up-to-date, self-righting lifeboat and felt happier after that day's training session. The lifeboat crew were excellent. They showed us all round and how to put on life jackets and what to do. With the training you feel more confident and now I would be pre-pared to go.

The helicopter is another story altogether. We haven't had training in helicopters. I understand ambulance personnel don't go in a helicopter because that isn't their remit. We're looking at that just now but again we would need to have training. One midwife had to put on a survival suit. She's very small and she looked like the Michelin man. She was told this was because they would be going over water and she might need to bale out. Another problem is, when the helicopter gets to its destination it doesn't bring you back because they have other things to do. So we then have to get a Health Board car to pick them up and bring them back. One of the midwives went out recently in what we called the 'yellow bug'. It's a little helicopter and there were the two crew, the midwife and the patient all very cramped together and she felt very unsafe. They've changed now to a slightly bigger one but we've also asked that that sort of thing be looked at for everybody's sake. The Trust need to make sure that the staff are happy and safe as well as the patients.

In our midwives' unit in Oban we make the decisions. We have a lot of autonomy. We change the service according to the patients' needs like the new midwives' clinic which has been such a success. Some things we cannot offer like epidurals and paediatric cover for ill babies. However, we feel we've moved with the times, possibly more than the bigger units because people ask questions about the service we provide and we stop and assess what we're doing.

Things have changed everywhere. Like perineal suturing – they aren't suturing so much now. Mothers come back from the consultant units with small tears and they aren't sutured. When you think about it, with a superficial perineal tear – you stand, walk, sit, and the wound isn't wide open. If you cut yourself you put the two pieces together so, why are we suturing them? It will come together naturally. The patients think it's wonderful.

I think the mothers probably have a nicer, more positive experience than before. Some people come to Oban especially to have a baby. One girl in particular whose sister lives in Oban came for a waterbirth . The GPs aren't happy with that because as far as they're concerned these patients are an unknown quantity and have had their antenatal care else-where. However, you can manage as long as they have a piece of paper with them with their antenatal history, or their 'Co-op card', or you can also phone their home unit and get further information.

There has been talk about stopping the night shift. This would affect me particularly. We went to a meeting at Fort William where they did away with the maternity unit night shift, partly because there are nights when they have no patients. That happened to me last week and I was on my own for ten hours. I do paperwork and things like that. In Fort William now a midwife sleeps in hospital every night and gets called if necessary and that could be a possibility.

If our numbers go up, we won't have to have that. At the moment the people are told there is a twenty-four-hour service, and some phone in the middle of the night with different problems. Some of them are health visitor calls, and some GP. If I can't help them I tell them either to contact their GP, or if it is advice about a baby over six weeks I might advise them to contact the health visitor in the morning. If I can, I give them advice over the phone and tell them to ring back if they still have a problem. If it's a crying baby, I sometimes suggest if they have transport that they bring the baby down here and I can check the baby over. Quite often by the time they're here the baby is asleep. Sometimes women come up at night, thinking they might be in labour. I check them over and send them home if they aren't in labour. They know we're there and arrive on the doorstep as in any maternity unit.

18

ALISON DALE
AND MAUREEN HAMILTON

Alison Dale and Maureen Hamilton trained as midwives in the late 1960s. Alison did Parts 1 and 2 of her training at the Maternity Hospital in Aberdeen and Maureen did Part 1 at a Maternity Hospital in England and Part 2 at Redlands Hospital in Glasgow. Currently, they both work as midwives in Aberdeen and here they discuss changes they have seen in maternity care.

ALISON I trained from August 1968 to August 1969 in Aberdeen. As well as the Maternity Hospital, there were maternity homes in Aberdeen: Summerfield, Queen's Cross and Fonthill. Summerfield, which was a big old house with additions, affiliated to the hospital, catered mostly for women with any antenatal problem needing long-term care like bleeding and habitual abortion. They'd twenty antenatal beds and women lay for the majority of their pregnancy. How they didn't all have DVTs I'll never know. They weren't even allowed up to the loo or to wash their hair. The head of the bed came off and they got their hair washed in bed. Twice a day they'd to lie down to sleep even though they didn't do anything else but rest. That was in the late 1960s and well into the 1970s.

MAUREEN I'm from Argyllshire and did Part 1 in England and returned to Glasgow and did Part 2 at Redlands, an old house made into a hospital and affiliated to Rotten Row, but very different. The training at Redlands left a lot to be desired. There was a lot of animosity and unhappiness there from sisters downwards.

157

The best bit was district. We were accepted everywhere, free transport on the buses and the subway and everybody thought the world of you. We were in uniform with our bag and there was no problem. I used to meet my midwife at Duke Street and do postnatal visits with her. When we were on night duty on the district we went to Ingram Street, near George Square, so that we could all be together. We sat in there all night, awake and in uniform, and waited. We were first on call, second on call etc., and when your midwife was called you went with her. If your midwife wasn't on that night you went with another midwife. A taxi came and took you to wherever you were going and brought you back after the delivery. We'd quite a few home deliveries and no problem getting them. After that [1969] the numbers went down.

ALISON There were very few home deliveries in Aberdeen by then. Only one girl in our set saw one. We went out on visits with the district midwife from our area and learned fast. One time, the husband was desperate for us to have a cup of tea and we said, 'No thanks'. When we went to wash our hands in the kitchen there were the soiled nappies and the dishes all in together.

There were about five, maybe six district midwives in the city. They had municipal housing and, I think, ran clinics from their houses. The ones I went with didn't have a car because they lived and worked in the area and didn't have to travel across the city. We walked or took the bus if we had to. During our Community Block we lived in, at Carden Place.

MAUREEN There was an awful storm in January 1968 and we went into this house off Duke Street. The three kids were all sitting watching the test-card on the TV in the sitting- room. In the bed-recess were mother, father and the new baby. The father got out of the bed fully clothed with a black suit, collar and tie, and said, 'Oh, we'll let you in to see the baby'. We dealt with the baby and he said, 'Come on through and see my storm damage', and in the kitchen there was a great hole in the middle of the floor. After that he went away out and left his wife and the baby and the three kids still sitting there watching the test-card.

One night, we went to Blackhill and delivered a woman. Her husband was involved with a gang and they were banging at the door while we were delivering the baby. He'd been involved in an attempted murder and some time later we read the story of him being charged in the evening paper. He was fine while we were there delivering his baby. We weren't frightened. I don't think you would find yourself in the same situation now.

ALISON I didn't have any home deliveries as a pupil midwife but I loved labour ward. That was where I wanted to be. In Part 2 we had to go to the milk kitchen, a little room in Ward Six of the Sick Children's Hospital, for a week. Babies were fed four-hourly whether they were asleep or not. They were advocating breastfeeding just like today, but there was a lot of formula feeding. We made up all the feeds for the wards and the prem-baby unit, wearing a gown, mask and gloves, on duty from 8a.m. till 5p.m. The feeds were made up from nine a.m. till two p.m. Then we collected in dirty bottles, and cleaned and sterilised them, all ready to start next day. They were narrow neck bottles with teats and little paper caps held on with rubber bands. It was hard going. The feeds were transported up to the Matty and kept in big fridges on the two floors.

In the Special Nursery we wore gown and mask most of the day. We'd two small isolation cubicles and that was it. Tiny little rooms. The ventilators were much bigger than they are now with a lot more piping and cylinders to be changed. The nursery was a much smaller unit and babies that are surviving now, just didn't survive then. Nobody would have thought about resuscitating a baby born at twenty-five weeks. If a baby was born at twenty-eight, twenty-nine weeks and went home you thought they were lucky. It's completely different now.

After qualifying as a midwife I went back to general

nursing for a year and then returned to midwifery. That was what I really wanted to do.

MAUREEN I returned to Campbeltown and worked in a GP Unit there for a year before getting married. We'd the Air Ambulance from Campbeltown to Glasgow if there were any complications. We also had a Flying Squad from the Southern General if there were complications and you couldn't move the mother.

Sometimes a GP, panicking, would say, 'Oh I think there are going to be problems. We'll need to get her to Glasgow'. Then she would deliver as soon as she arrived. If the Air Ambulance was in use we accompanied the mother to the airport and handed her over to a midwife from Glasgow. We didn't have many deliveries. You could go a couple of weeks with none and then we might have about five so I don't know how many there were in a year. We'd the mothers postnatally and they loved it. They stayed in hospital for about seven days then and it was a real home from home for them, overlooking the loch. It was good if they could deliver there. The GPs weren't that keen to get involved but seemed delighted to come and find the mother delivered and everything fine. The midwife still did the delivery when the GP was there, but it was only very occasionally they were. You phoned them to say Mrs So-and-So was in but they only came if you were in difficulties. They would say, 'Give me a shout if you need me'. It was very different from working in Aberdeen with labour ward along the corridor from the midwives' unit to give back-up.

ALISON Fonthill was lovely if everything was straightforward but if you'd a complication in the rush-hour Fonthill was a long way away from the Matty. If you'd shoulder dystocia or a flat baby in the middle of the night, help could be there in four or five minutes which is still a long time, but if they got caught up in the rush-hour it could maybe be twelve or fourteen minutes before help arrived and that's a *very* long time.

Alison Dale and Maureen Hamilton

MAUREEN I don't think people realise if they haven't worked outwith a unit like Aberdeen how frightening it can be. In Campbeltown we'd a very experienced sister who lived in. Even if she wasn't on duty, if there was a problem and you called her she never minded. You always knew she was there.

ALISON That was similar to the system in the Homes in Aberdeen. Whichever sister had been on duty during the day slept in overnight and you could call on her if necessary. However, at Fonthill, Miss Madge Archibald lived in a flat at the top. If there was a problem you just phoned or knocked on her door and she'd come down. If someone needed to be transferred, the midwife looking after her would go with her and the one sleeping in would oversee until she came back.

ALISON Aberdeen, in the late 1960s, was quite medicalised. Midwives at that time didn't make any decisions. Medical staff made the decision and the midwife just did as she was told. We didn't know any different. Very much the hand-maiden to the consultants. The consultants did a ward round and everybody followed on behind them with everything ready for them. You'd be asked questions about your patients and were expected to know the answer. Then things began to change. We began to involve the mother and say, 'I think we should maybe let this woman try a wee bit longer', or to the woman, 'What would *you* like, Mrs So-and-So?'

MAUREEN I noticed when I came back to work in 1980 there was quite a change from the late sixties. It was definitely more woman centred then. They were asked their opinions and they were told everything, from start to finish. If the baby was in the Nursery, they weren't kept in the dark about anything.

ALISON Even in the 1970s things were still very medically orientated and parents just visited, they weren't told every-thing and they didn't like to ask many questions. Only parents were allowed to visit whether the baby was in the Nursery for three days or three months. Grandparents never saw the baby. In the 1980s people became less frightened to ask. Patients lost their fear of the consultant and the medical staff. People found they had an input into what concerned them and they could challenge. The media helped, people became more able and they weren't frightened to say, 'Excuse me, I don't agree with you,' or, 'Why are you doing that?'

MAUREEN They were encouraged at antenatal classes as well, to say what they wanted

ALISON Yes. Antenatal classes probably really changed in the eighties. It wasn't just what *we* decided any more. The mothers became very well-read and more vociferous. They developed a lot of insight. Midwives too responded to the challenge, spoke up for the mothers and stopped being apprehensive of the doctors. They would ask the mum, 'What do you think? What would you like?' and get her to give her opinion.

MAUREEN I think doctors probably have more respect for midwives now than they had before. Now they accept that you are a practitioner and hopefully you know what you're talking about. Certainly they listen to us a lot more.

ALISON Yes, and so do the young SHOs, who come to obstetrics knowing very little. They seem happy to get a midwife in with them and ask if they are doing something right.

ALISON I got back to the labour ward in the early 1970s. I worked in the labour ward for about three or four months on day duty and then we were getting married so, if you worked night duty you got extra money, so I did about ten months on labour ward nights and thoroughly enjoyed it.

Now, I do about sixteen hours a week in antenatal clinic and about eight hours in the community. That includes an antenatal clinic on Wednesday afternoon and one on a Thursday morning, both at surgeries, and then I do antenatal and postnatal visits.

Alison Dale and Maureen Hamilton

To get back to the labour ward in the 1970s – they did the inductions in the evening then, so the nights were busy. Induction was done by ARM and if the mothers didn't go into labour they had intravenous Syntocinon started. We still had the old antenatal ward then. They came in there and they were examined vaginally. Then they came round to Labour Ward, had their membranes ruptured and returned to the antenatal ward. When they started contracting, they came back to the labour ward. This procedure went on for quite a while and we were very busy.

We've really come a long way since then. We don't do archaic things like shaving our mothers now. They would be horrified if we said we were going to shave them. So it's a lot better than it was. There was far too much intervention. I think a lot of people think that in the North-east, there are a lot of social inductions because of offshore workers. I don't think there is. There were social inductions a few years ago but now that is right down at the bottom of the queue.

They can do five inductions per day, and inductions for medical reasons take priority. Post-mature mothers go up to term plus fourteen days and sometimes it's difficult giving them a date for induction and sticking to it, because of possible emergencies. We warn them about this. The same happens to mothers booked for an elective section. If there were an emergency, an elective section might have to be put off till the next day.

In the 1970s they also had the stabilising induction. This was if the mother had an unstable lie. She had her ARM with someone holding the fetal head head down at the pelvis. Hopefully there would be loads of liquor so the baby's head would go down. However, this poor woman was not allowed to move. She was propped up on lots of pillows supporting her sitting upright until the fetal head was well into the pelvis and you could guarantee that you wouldn't have a prolapsed cord.

These were the days before epidurals when you'd all the back-rubbing especially with OP. You had these poor girls with these long drawn-out labours. Again there were a lot of pillows involved, to keep them round on their side. I can still feel my fist on the sacrum to help the backache in the OP position.

Husbands were not encouraged in the labour ward but got in if they wanted. Nobody else. No partners! Nor mothers. The first time I had a husband there, he landed on the floor! Even if they phoned to ask about their wife, we weren't all that pleased. They would come in and drop the wife off and say, 'I'll phone back'. I remember this chap brought his wife in. They already had one child and she was huge with what turned out to be undiagnosed twins. The husband phoned late at night and he was told he had twins and the phone went dead. About half an hour later he arrived and said, 'I got a message but I think it was wrong. My wife came in only to have one baby'. The poor lad. He was a joiner and he came in the next day with a tape measure measuring the cribs we had. He was going to make a cot that would take the two babies.

Husbands only saw their baby at visiting time. We'd a chap in quite recently whose second wife was having a baby. He told us that when his first wife was having their second baby in the mid-1970s he was working offshore. He was sent for and arrived at about half-past-eight in the evening. His wife had had the baby and he wasn't allowed in because it was past visiting time. It just shows how things have changed in twenty years. Now husbands, partners are there almost twenty-four hours a day.

MAUREEN They're there all day except from twelve till two-thirty when the women have their lunch and their afternoon sleep, and when they have their tea. In the evening they're there till half-past-nine. It's quite a lot really. The mothers get too tired.

ALISON I think it's all the other visitors too.

MAUREEN Also when they're breastfeeding, it's not easy when visitors are around especially when some of the girls are struggling a bit.

Alison Dale and Maureen Hamilton

ALISON In the seventies we used to take all the babies out to the nursery at night and the mums got a sleep. They weren't popular if they said they wanted to keep their baby beside them. Now the babies are with the mothers all the time. I think that's probably why they go home much sooner.

MAUREEN They also go home sooner, when there are other children. They don't get a break at all.

MAUREEN When I came back to work on the midwives' bank in 1980, to begin with I worked anywhere in the unit. I found I'd lost my confidence in labour ward and it was quite frightening. On the bank you only go to labour ward if it's busy and don't get enough time there to build up your confidence, especially if you've been away from work for a while. As things developed I worked mostly in the scan department and very occasionally going to different places. Now I work in the scan department all the time and they tell me when they need me in advance. I was happier working with antenatal women. I've always preferred this. I love it. I work now in the day-ward within the scan department and it's all antenatals, amniocentesis, CVS, CTGs, breakfast test meals and any tests that the mothers can come in for and go home. I still like postnatal and I enjoy the neonatal unit.

In the Day Ward, the hours are 8.30am till 5pm. If a mother has diabetes, or a suspected big baby, or anything else making us suspect diabetes like elevated random blood glucose, the mother comes to us and we do a breakfast test meal. It's the same idea as a glucose tolerance test but she's with us for the whole morning. We take blood first and then we give her breakfast of Complan and three digestive biscuits, and two hours after that we take more blood from her. She gets tea and toast after that. There are often about four mothers in having this and they talk together about their children and so on. This can be the start of quite a good rapport between them as they usually meet up again at other appointments.

If anybody goes to their GP or their community midwife and they have reduced fetal movements, they phone and they come to us for a CTG tracing and a Doppler scan. That's all done in the department so it's quite a busy place. You don't know what's going to happen next as they can come at any time. Mothers come from the clinics as well for CTG tracings and mothers with thyroid and diabetic problems come for tracings when they come to the combined clinic. It's a nice unit to work in. I really enjoy it. There's only one midwife in the ward and an auxiliary – called an outpatient assistant.

We're within the scan department where there are another two or three midwives scanning. They're all trained in scanning and are very good. Some of them have done a Diploma in Ultrasound as well. There are also radiographers scanning. The midwives are best with the mothers as it's their speciality and they understand better. The mums say that they find the midwives more approachable because they know more about this specific subject.

We do amniocentesis as well. We've also started doing ECVs, external cephalic version, again. Turning the babies *in utero* stopped for a long time but they're doing it again in Aberdeen. One particular consultant attempts ECVs here. The mother has a CTG first and then he scans her to see exactly what is happening. Then he attempts to turn the baby gently. He says to them beforehand what it will entail and he has no intention of hurting them and they must say if it's too much for them. If the baby is not likely to turn, or if it's too painful for the mum, he stops right away. He scans them again and brings them back through to the ward and we do another CTG to make sure the baby is all right. If all's well they go home. If the baby hasn't turned they come back to their clinic appointment the following week and their own consultant will have a chat with them about delivery. It's by no means a foregone conclusion that they need a Caesarean section.

He's very good with them and has had a lot of successes. The women who are Rhesus Negative get Anti-D when they have it done just in case. I think the overall success rate for ECVs at Aberdeen is about forty percent.

Alison Dale and Maureen Hamilton

ALISON The ECV isn't attempted before thirty-seven weeks. I don't know if the rate of breech deliveries has gone up. It depends on the mother and we've quite a few girls who say that they will give breech delivery a try. However, if she doesn't want to try, then she can have a section. The current theory is that there is no definite advantage to the babies who are breech presentation being delivered by CS. We used to think there was, but now they don't think so and they're compiling a lot of statistics on the issue.

MAUREEN If they get the baby turned at thirty-seven weeks he doesn't usually turn back. We've had the odd one. The medical staff deliver breeches in theatre.

A lot of antenatal care is done on the community if everything is straightforward. Even if mothers are referred for one hospital visit they normally go back out into the community. Even when the girls were having treatment from the fertility unit, once they're pregnant, if possible they should have care in the community.

ALISON 'Tucker' is a new system of care which was supposed to be all over Scotland. The instigators of Tucker was our Dr Hall and Dr Frances Tucker. She now works three days a week in the Dugald Baird Unit. With Tucker, if everything is straightforward whether prims or parous patients, they can have their care in the community. That's midwife and GP or just midwife, depending on what the system is at the surgery. They'll only have two visits to the hospital, one for a booking scan and one for a detailed anomaly scan at twenty weeks. All the rest of the care will be done in the community. Even if they go past their dates, the community midwife will phone into the Queen's Cross Unit where we do our inductions. They're allocated a consultant, so if there's a problem, they can be referred.

If a mother has any previous medical problem if they're prims, or any previous obstetric or medical problem if they're parous, they have shared care. For example, previous sections, previous stillbirth, previous PPH, are all classed as

requiring shared care, that is hospital and community. However, they only have a first visit to see the consultant or one of
the team and if all's well, they're looked after by the community staff and referred back if there's a problem. In one of
the surgeries where I do a clinic, the midwife sees all the
patients there. The GPs have very little input. If there's a
problem we send the mother to the Matty. Things are
changing all the time. For reduced fetal movements we used
to need a CTG tracing. Now the criteria for fetal wellbeing
have been changed and they're doing Doppler for fetal wellbeing far more than CTG. A Doppler scan gives a better
prognosis for a few days whereas a CTG will only inform
about the current situation. The Doppler's where you can
look at the bloodflow, the endiastolic flow through the
bloodvessels, and it shows up on a graph on the scanning
machine.

Mothers who are straightforward don't need to be seen at
the hospital. However, they get to know their midwife well
but they don't have her for the delivery. If they're going to
have a DOMINO they'll have one of the team but if they're
having a hospital confinement they don't know who's going
to deliver them. I think that's a problem but how do you get
round it?

We've a Midwives' Unit and in it look after mothers
who're straightforward. Mothers booked for Tucker – community care, and the ones with least visits to the hospital
antenatally – are all booked for the Midwives' Unit. When in
the Midwives' Unit, if there's a problem, or if a mother
decides she wants an epidural, she's moved to the consultant
unit. Mothers for shared care are normally booked for the
obstetric unit unless the reason is something very insignif-
icant.

MAUREEN They make it as near home as possible. They use a
Pinard's stethoscope and Sonicaid for listening into the fetal
heart and that's all.

ALISON There's very little interference at all.

Alison Dale and Maureen Hamilton

MAUREEN No medical staff.

ALISON But if there's a problem they can go along the corridor and they're in labour ward.

MAUREEN The doctors can come in if there's a problem and if they're invited – asked to come and see someone.

ALISON The midwives like working there. The midwives in Labour Ward rotate through to the Midwives' Unit.

MAUREEN I think they do it for four weeks at a time.

ALISON If a mother's having a DOMINO, she'll come into the Midwives' Unit with her community midwife. And then we have the bath – the birthing-pool. It's used a lot, particularly for pain relief in labour but not so much for delivery.

MAUREEN It was trendy for a while. We'd quite a few water-births and there was a lot of publicity but now most mothers seem to like the bath when they're in labour, for pain-relief, but come out to deliver.

ALISON It takes a good forty-five minutes to fill the bath. It takes a terrific amount of water. It's a huge bath.

19

JOAN SPENCE

Joan Spence trained as a midwife in Aberdeen in 1970. Since then, she has practised as a midwife in Aberdeen, Australia and Edinburgh. She is currently Head of Midwifery in the Maternity Unit in Borders General Hospital and is working on a project to create an integrated midwifery service for the Borders.

I decided to be a midwife when I was working as a nursery nurse in Thornhill Maternity Unit in Paisley. The midwives there were very good and would let me into the labour suite to watch deliveries. I had to train as a nurse first as direct entry to midwifery in Scotland had just stopped. Otherwise I think I would have gone straight into midwifery. So I did my general nurse training at the Victoria Infirmary in Glasgow and when I qualified a group of us went straight up to Aberdeen to do midwifery. It was a year's training and I thoroughly enjoyed it.

I did my training in 1970, staffed in the nursery which I enjoyed, then I did the four months' neonatal course. I particularly remember the first baby to be ventilated on an adult ventilator and the high number of abnormal babies which, because we didn't have scans, were undiagnosed before birth. There were babies with deformities of their limbs and microcephaly. There always seemed to be abnormal babies in the nursery. I think that's why the staff take it so hard now because they don't see it so often.

We had only been qualified about two years when five of us were told we were going to be Sisters. The Salmon re-organisation came in 1974 and some very experienced ward sisters were shunted out to walk the corridors as Nursing

170

Officers. I didn't feel ready for a sister's post but was told that if I didn't do it I would never get another one. When I got used to it, I felt very comfortable in Special Care and the postnatal ward where I was working.

After about nine months, the 'change-list' announced that I was going to labour ward as a sister. I didn't have much experience here but again I was told I had to go. The staff midwives there had more experience than I had but nobody seemed to mind. I particularly remember night duty. They knew I was quite raw and they were so kind and taught me so much. After a while I calmed down, gained confidence and enjoyed it. But it wasn't the best way to learn. They don't do that to people nowadays.

It was very regimented. The labour ward had five or six delivery rooms. At the top of it we had a little two-bedded first-stage room. Very often the labour rooms were full, there were women in this first-stage room and women labouring in the antenatal ward. Quite often they would come round on a bed and deliver in the corridor.

Induction was the in thing. They did away with the two-bedded first-stage room and they built on an induction suite. We admitted about eight women every evening about 8pm. They all had their waters broken then and usually half of them would go into labour. If you were on night duty you knew you would have three or four labouring women from this group and anyone else who arrived in spontaneous labour. In the morning the four who were not in labour came round and had Syntocinon drips up. They were delivered by four in the afternoon. The rates of Syntocinon in Aberdeen were enormous. We were taught as student midwives how to build up a regime, doubling the units up to about 164 units of Syntocinon. The midwives were trained to monitor the contractions and know when the uterus could or could not take more. Looking back, it was a scary business. But you didn't know any different then.

I don't think mothers were given any option. They were all in bed and there was no walking about. They were starved apart from glucose boiled sweeties. Also, if a woman had been in labour a long time or if labour had stopped, they got this disgusting blended food called Tormix, which they didn't like, to keep them going. It was almost like stovies or potato and gravy put through the blender. They were starved from the minute they were induced or they came in in labour.

I remember when epidurals were introduced and then we had a twenty-four hour epidural service. One night they couldn't get epidurals. It wasn't until we didn't have them that I remembered what it had been like before. With those high levels of Syntocinon the women needed maximum pain relief. Without it they were screaming all over the place. We also used Pethilorfan and Pethidine.

At the time Aberdeen, for some reason, had a very high rate of pre-eclampsia. PIH as it is nowadays. They had a very unique, complicated regime of drugs to deal with that and an equally complicated system of administering these drugs and trying to cut down the patient's fluids through a Palmer pump. One of the first things you learned as a midwife in the labour ward was how to set the pump up.

We had a lot of normal deliveries but also many doctors around linked with university teaching. We had a good relationship with the doctors. There was always a good atmosphere. We had quite good fun in the labour ward although night duty was horrendous. There were many more midwives on during the day than at night. You would come on at night and there was probably the sister, two part-time staff midwives, a couple of student midwives and that was it. And all these patients coming hurtling through the door. I can remember one night in particular giving the handover in the morning and I had this big pile of case-notes and some of the patients I hadn't seen. I can remember having thirteen, fourteen admissions sometimes on night duty in the labour ward with maybe three or four of you on.

A big difference nowadays is the way they handle still-births. We didn't know, we thought we were doing the right thing – whipping these babies away . Wrapping them up, out the door and the mother never saw it again. We didn't do it maliciously. We did it because we thought that was the best way. One day, a lady was rushed round from antenatal on a bed, delivering. She had two little boys already and the head was there and because I didn't have time to get a student, I delivered the baby myself. It was always nice to get your hands on to a baby. The wee chap came out and he was grossly deformed. His limbs were all round the wrong way. I ran out of the room with him and I ran into a paediatrician. The baby was barely alive. The paediatrician wanted to take him from me and resuscitate him but he died within minutes. That poor woman, I've never forgotten her. I don't think she ever saw that baby again. She would have nightmares wondering what he looked like, and it would have been so much easier just to let her see. His face was OK . The reality would have been better than what she was imagining.

Women were very accepting of the care that they got and didn't question. They came in, did what they were told and went home again. Then I see the women here today and their labours are so much better. They are well, and the pain-relief is so good. They're up the next day and away home. When I think back, some of these women were quite debilitated by the whole experience. You saw them in the postnatal ward and they looked shell-shocked, especially the prims. We were kind to them but I don't think the psychological side of it was explored. We didn't sit down and debrief them in any way about the labour. It was all physical. We're much better at the psychological side now. Also, the women are much better prepared. They're more interested antenatally and they ask questions.

The postnatal ward has changed. I remember as a student, we took all these blessed babies into the big nursery and they cried all night and we stuck bottles in them. Now peace reigns. There is the odd wee whimper and the baby will either be put to the breast or the mother bottlefeeds him. We had thirty-odd babies in this room all crying. I suppose the mother got a good night's sleep. We weren't doing things to be bad. We were doing them because we thought it was right. Then women started to say, 'I don't think this is right. No, I want my baby with me all night. I'm not going to carry a baby with me for nine months and then give it to you to take away to a nursery'.

I went to Australia in 1978 and I was away for four years. When I came back I did the health visitor course and then worked as a health visitor for a few months. I enjoyed the course but I wasn't too keen on being a health visitor. A vacancy occurred for a Nursing Officer type post for the Western General in Edinburgh covering SCBU and the Post-natal Ward. I applied for it, got the job and moved down to Edinburgh.

The Maternity Unit at the Western was lovely. So small after Aberdeen – quite similar to here. They had about twelve hundred deliveries a year. The building was decrepit but the care was good and the midwives were excellent. They were all similar, kind, gentle midwives and it was a lovely unit. I really felt I had come home when I got to the Western.

Active childbirth started. I remember the very first lady who came in. I came on one morning and the sister who had been on night duty in the labour ward had tears running down her cheeks laughing. She said, 'I've got this lady in and and she's jogging round the admission room. She wants active childbirth'. The lady had on a nightie and she had red socks and she was determined she was going to keep UPRIGHT. She was literally jogging round the admission room. That was the start. The women started to come in saying, 'I don't want to lie down. I want to walk about. I don't want to deliver on the bed. I want to deliver on a mattress on the floor'. To begin with it was all very odd. We all thought, what's all this about? But the midwives there were very good and flexible and even the older ones had enough experience to say, 'Well, let's give it a go'.

The WRVS decided they would buy us a birthing chair. It was an awful-looking thing but this was the latest thing. It was a hydraulic thing and it looked like a dentist's chair. So we got this birthing chair but it didn't last very long because the women's perineums suffered. We delivered a few but it cost four and a half thousand pounds at the time. Then we got bean-bags and mattresses on the floor and so on and the women started to write out birth plans.

That was really the way it started and then came babies rooming-in. I can remember the fuss the obstetric consultants made about this. What on earth were they doing putting the babies into the wards? The babies usually came in and out for feeding. We pushed them in and pulled them out. First thing in the morning they were all lined up. They all got topped and tailed at the same time, instead of being done beside their mums. They weren't bathed beside their mums either.

Anyway we decided we would give this a go. We had all read and become quite knowledgeable about rooming-in and the sister in the ward was excellent and keen to do it. The sister was really into breastfeeding in a big way and had an excellent rapport with the women. We had a ten-bedded postnatal room, a little three-bedded room for sections and a twelve bedded room. I said to her, 'Look, let's just put the babies out in the ten-bedded room and see if the consultants even notice'. They were creating such a fuss about it. So we put them out for a week and nobody said anything. So then we put them all out. The next time one of the consultants said, 'What about this rooming-in?' I said,'Oh it's been happening for a fortnight'. So that was it. Done. These issues were purely midwifery. The consultants were lovely people at the Western and easy to work with. But really rooming-in was a midwife's decision. Nowadays they would say,'Why are you asking me? That's *your* job'.

I left the Western in 1988 because a Head of Midwifery post came up at the Eastern General Hospital in Edinburgh. It was a similar-sized unit, slightly bigger. It was a very progressive little unit, taking forward quite a lot of issues. Again they had active childbirth, birth plans, women doing their own thing.

Breastfeeding was encouraged. The Western closed not long after I left. The staff were all deployed round Edinburgh and some of them came to the Eastern. I took the opportunity of having an extra sister from the postnatal ward to have a breastfeeding sister. I acknowledge that breastfeeding is every midwife's remit.However, I don't think it does any harm to have somebody who is an expert in that. She took on the role of breastfeeding adviser and she also homed in on all these families who had special problems or needs like parents of little babies in SCBU or single mums. Sandra was amazing with them. Once they were discharged, she visited them at home just to make sure that things were fine. One single mother in particular had a lot of problems. Sandra did some parenthood education with her and mothered her a bit. After she got home with her little boy she returned quite often to see us. About a month before the child's first birthday she came in and said, 'It's his first birthday coming up and I can't make up my mind what to do on that day. It's a toss-up between taking him to the zoo or bringing him to the Eastern for his birthday'. I thought, we're going to end up having all the children coming back for their birthdays. A day out at the Eastern. On the day we had a wee party for her with a cake. Sandra gave her and so many others such a lot of support. The midwives in the ward always dealt with the breastfeeders but if they had anyone with particular difficulties, Sandra was brought in to give some advice and help. Now, money is so tight that these posts are few and far between.

In 1994 I came down here as Director of Midwifery for the whole of the Borders. This was as a result of the work of the Maternity Services Liaison Group which was set up in the Borders in the early 1990s. Lady Sanderson was the chairman. She produced their report saying that the way forward was to integrate the service. On the strength of that they appointed me.

However, I was only here about nine months when the Government decided the Borders Health Service should be divided into two Trusts – one community, and one a hospital Trust, with community midwives in one Trust and me in the other. So my job disappeared. I ended up having the maternity unit here and all the surgical wards and orthopaedics. So the maternity unit was in the surgical directorate of which I was the senior nurse/midwife. I hadn't been a nurse since I had been a student nurse and I finished in 1969. This really was not why I came to the Borders. At the same time SCBU and the Nursery and the children's ward were put into the medical directorate. These changes set integration of mid-wifery in the Borders back about four years. The Report was put on the back burner and no matter how much complaining I did, it was done.

We were re-organised again in July 1999 and they took surgical and orthopaedics away from me. Now they've put maternity, SCBU, the children's ward and gynaecology all back together again. So that's what I have now. Community is still now a Primary Care Trust with the community mid-wives doing double-duty, and some treble-duty. However, we have moved on and the Health Board wrote specifications for maternity and midwifery services in about August-September 1999 which they put to the two Trusts. It was for an integrated service.

The two Trusts got together at my level and the DNS level and we put a paper together, put a bid into the Health Board asking for enough money to second a project leader for a year into the community – a G grade level person – to work with community midwives at a clinical level for half the time to see what their problems were. The other half of this person's time would be spent looking at the service, how to bring the two services together and what sort of model of care we would need to provide.

There's an area in the central Borders round the hospital like Galashiels, Melrose, Selkirk, probably up as far as Ear-lston and Lauder where you could have a truly integrated service with midwives working in and out of the unit. The rest is too far from the unit. Eyemouth is a long way away from Melrose, West Linton is nearly in Lanarkshire, New-castleton is nearer Carlisle than it is here. We would need to look at a different model for those areas. To our delight the Health Board said they would fund this person to go out.

I think the central Borders area could have maybe one team of midwives to look after the women who live there wherever the woman is, either hospital or at home. The same team of midwives would give her care throughout pregnancy, labour and postnatal. In and out I would hope. The farther out areas will need a different idea. One of the G-grade midwives in the unit has been doing a project on teams. We have four consultants who each have a geographical area in which they do peripheral clinics. We thought we could maybe have a team of midwives for each of those. When the women come in they would have that team to look after them for labour and postnatally. So, for the far-flung areas, we could have the teams in the hospital and have a link midwife to the community midwives in the area. One of the big problems is helping community midwives come in to update their skills. If we had a link midwife in each team who could go out and do a day out in the community, the community midwife could come in and spend a day here, or something like that. She could come and do an antenatal clinic in here with the clinic sister and update on all the latest screening.

We also held an evening session recently on home births because we have quite a few home births. I think we had thirteen last year, quite a lot for a total of a thousand deliveries. One of the community midwives had asked for an update on home births, and one of our new consultants – it was really more on obstetric emergencies – said he would be happy to do an evening session. We held this session here and more community midwives than we imagined appeared. They said it was super and could we not have more? So we're hoping to try and get more of that type of thing. Also some of the hospital midwives were there too, so it has brought the two camps together.

We have also had a working group of hospital and community midwives working on different protocols and procedures. We've just changed the on-call recently. All the on-call comes through the labour ward now. Before, the community midwives had to do their ordinary on-call plus the home births on call. So all women now get a leaflet, and if they want advice or help they contact the labour ward. There's a midwife there twenty-four hours a day who can easily give advice. Most of the time the mothers need reassurance and somebody at the end of a phone. The midwife always says, 'Phone me back in an hour and let me know how you are getting on'. This takes the pressure off the community midwife. The midwives here are up and awake and could be on the phone all night to them if they want.

The hospital and community working groups work very well together. Occasionally there are times when each group feels the other lot doesn't understand the individual problems. We're working on that – trying to get them to understand each other's predicament. If we can start getting midwives out of here, into the community, and bring the others in, then they'll start to appreciate each other's role better. On the community it's quite frightening to be all alone in the middle of nowhere and responsible.

So, hopefully in the next year we're going to be taking the service forward further than I had ever envisaged. At least it will be well started before I retire. We will have to go gently and take everybody's feelings into account. You can't just put people out of a job because we're changing. At least we'll have plans in place for what we think is the best model for a midwifery service for the Borders. Hopefully we'll be starting this in 2000. I'm amazed. I never thought it would happen. It's all really because the Health Board have had the foresight to give us the money because we couldn't have done it otherwise.

We have already implemented single-duty midwifery in Hawick and Jedburgh. It happened when they had vacancies. Instead of putting in district nurse/midwives, we put in staff nurses to do the nursing part and midwives for the midwifery. We have one part-time and two full-time midwives in Hawick and Jedburgh. That's the only place in the Borders where that has happened. It works OK but they're on a shoestring with no relief cover.

The community management did well seizing the opportunity in Jedburgh and Hawick. The GPs didn't want any change but now they're very happy. They can see that these midwives are very skilled and that they, the GPs, can let go a little bit and concentrate on other things. They see that the women are getting a good deal. From our point of view, communication is easier with these midwives because we're all talking the same language. I would say it will take five years to get it going completely.

We have a super little unit here. We all have our strengths and weaknesses but the midwives here are so enthusiastic and so committed and wanting to push out the boundaries. They really want women to get what they should get. For instance we have a lovely birthing pool room here now. It's lovely to work with people like that. It's wonderful to have such back-up – people on the staff where you can say, 'Let's try such and such. What do you think?' and they'll say, 'That's a good idea. Let's try it'. It makes life so much easier. The job becomes a pleasure when you have people who're pushing out the boundaries.

20

RAIGMORE MIDWIVES: AYLEEN MARSHALL, NIKKI MORTON, GRETA RENWICK, JOAN KELLY

Four midwives working at the Maternity Unit in Raigmore Hospital, Inverness, discuss maternity care in Inverness including team midwifery, waterbirths and problems of caring for mothers in Raigmore's wide catchment area in the Highlands of Scotland.

JOAN Here in Raigmore we have evolved a method of team midwifery with four teams. Midwives are assigned to a team and work within the unit but not out into the community. There are usually two midwives of varying grades and experience on duty per team at a time.

AYLEEN Each team has a team leader who is a G grade midwife.

JOAN Each team functions as a unit, in which the sister can decide what she wants her team members to do, and the teams can decide how they want to function and how much responsibility for managing the team they want to take.

AYLEEN A mother is allocated to a team antenatally so that she'll meet her team midwives before she goes into labour. Theoretically, she should know the midwife looking after her in labour but this also depends on staffing levels
Midwives work in the wards or labour suite although we base a member from each team in labour ward for a month at

a time to try and help develop our skills and extend our experience. This also helps team staffing levels. Sometimes they're quite stretched if we have too many mothers from the same team in labour at the same time.

JOAN Sometimes you can go for a week or a fortnight without being in labour suite, and if you're trying to get your suturing skills up to date it's quite difficult to keep the momentum going.

NIKKI When I finished my training at Ayrshire Central in March 1998 they offered me eighteen hours a week at D grade which I didn't want, whereas Wick was advertising full-time E grade posts. Wick is a small unit where you do a bit of everything and operates like team midwifery. There are two labour rooms, and although there are only 250 deliveries a year, it was good experience. After a year there, I came here. To be really confident in labour suite, I would like at least six months there. When you're there for your month, by the end you are just starting to feel comfortable when you're back working as a member of the team.

GRETA This is a disadvantage of team midwifery. I'm newly qualified – in March 1999 – and I also would like to be based in labour suite for longer. During my training I felt we didn't get enough clinical time, especially in labour suite. As a midwife I would have been happy to rotate round the departments in the unit every six months to give me confidence.

NIKKI Maybe it would be a good idea for midwives when they're newly qualified to rotate for a year before going into the teams.

AYLEEN When I qualified I went to work in Dr Gray's Hospital, Elgin for four months with no team midwifery and no midwifery students. I could be in labour ward whenever I wanted and got good experience. After I came back to Raigmore I was lucky at one point to work in the labour ward for six months.

JOAN I think all newly qualified midwives should go straight into labour suite for six months, and get all their labour ward skills up to date before going to the wards. Morale would improve, midwives would feel more confident, and with happier midwives the system is more likely to work. We shouldn't underestimate the amount to be learned on the wards too. Running a busy ward can be just as demanding.

GRETA Rotation seems to have gone out of fashion, which is a pity. Through my training, the emphasis was on the midwife being able to do everything. If we could concentrate in one area, it would take eighteen months to get through the three areas, but that would be better than eighteen months of trying to learn everything all at once.

JOAN Don't forget the benefits to women with team midwifery. It can be very worthwhile to be able to give a woman continuity of care from start to finish. I recently got a card from a lady I delivered. I was on for three days and on the first day I looked after her antenatally. We talked about her plans to have her baby adopted and the next day I delivered her baby. She wanted to breastfeed the baby and that was fine. Some people thought she should not have breastfed when she was going to have the baby adopted. But it was her baby and if she wanted to breastfeed, then that was her privilege.

The next day I spent a lot of time with her. The ward was quiet and there was time to talk. When I had to leave, she still had the baby with her and I got the impression that she wasn't going to let him go. I asked her to let me know how she got on and she sent me a picture of her baby on his first birthday. She had decided against adoption. I didn't pressurise her in any way. I was just there for her and that is how the teams can give continuity. She could have had three different midwives looking after her. Each of the three midwives could have done the same job as me but the continuity that's there is important.

Scottish Midwives

NIKKI It's good to be able to care for someone from before she goes into labour right through labour and the birth into the postnatal period. I think the mothers who have been looked after like that feel very satisfied by the time they go home.

AYLEEN The girls who have been looked after with problems during the latter weeks of pregnancy get to know their team midwives individually and *we* get to know *them* so well.

We don't usually go out into the community but one day when I was based on labour ward, one of the community midwives was off sick. I went to help them out and visited four mothers I had delivered over the previous few days. It was a very enjoyable experience and would be good for us to be able to do more often. You see the mothers in a whole different light.

NIKKI Grading is a problem in midwifery. Here there is very little promotion to F grade. In Wick I was one of two E grades. All the other midwives up there were F grades.

GRETA I was sent to Wick as my first placement during my training here for about eight weeks and really enjoyed it. They were so helpful and keen for us to learn. We stayed in the Nurses' Home and they would phone us there if someone came in. When I returned for my next placement it was a huge culture shock. It was so different.

NIKKI People told me that Wick was not the best place to go when you're newly qualified because it's such a small unit. However, for me the transition from student to staff midwife in Wick was great because even if we did sometimes only have three patients we didn't sit in the office and ignore them. You could sit with them and give them parentcraft and talk to them about labour.

AYLEEN Wick, unlike Raigmore, probably has a problem recruiting staff because it's quite far away. So it does have to pay them.

Raigmore Midwives

NIKKI It does, but that shouldn't be. When I had been there four months as a newly qualified midwife and one of three E grades there at the time, they had a vacancy for an F grade midwife. The sister said, 'I hope you will all apply for this post'. She pointed out that we were doing the same job. They employed us as E grades but they expected once we had learned how to manage the ward including transferring patients to Raigmore that we should be upgraded.

The problem of paying midwives could maybe be dealt with like medical staff. You could have junior, middle and senior midwives.

JOAN Grading really stunts midwives' professional development, and is partly responsible for low morale.

NIKKI You could either change the system or automatically become an F grade when somebody leaves.

JOAN In other areas of the UK you will be given an F grade after six months of taking up an E grade post, on reaching competency in cannulation, suturing and other labour suite skills.

GRETA One of my class moved to Kent, got a permanent post immediately and was told at interview she would have six months to become competent at suturing and venepuncture. Once that was achieved she would become an F grade.

AYLEEN It's good for us to have total care of a woman in normal labour and postnatally. She won't need to see anybody else. But it isn't very encouraging for me, qualified for two years, to see someone who has been qualified for eleven years and being paid the same grade as I am. I've completed my degree since I qualified and I sometimes wonder why I bothered.

JOAN I've done the Advanced Diploma in Midwifery and am working for my degree too.

Scottish Midwives

AYLEEN: You wonder why you put money, time and effort into doing extra qualifications when you're not going to be promoted. But, on the other hand, it's important with litigation to keep up-to-date with current research and policies.

JOAN One of our colleagues told us about someone on television who said, 'Midwives are not in it for the money. It's a vocation'. I think most midwives do it because we enjoy it. You can't look after a woman in labour and build up a relationship if you don't enjoy what you're doing. You're trying to give them a good experience but you also benefit.

NIKKI That comes back to feeling confident in labour suite. If I'm in a room, looking after a woman, and everything is normal and I've done everything for her, it's very enjoyable. If I can do everything by myself without asking for help I come away feeling great. Probably so does the mother because she has confidence in me. It isn't good enough to have to ask somebody to suture for me because I'm not getting the experience.

JOAN I think you have to push yourself to gain this. But, you can lose your skills. I was off on maternity leave. When I came back, I had to re-learn.

AYLEEN We're quite lucky here in that we have a lot of midwives who are very competent. It's only since I came back here from Elgin that I gained suturing experience.

NIKKI It's a good thing for a woman to be able to choose her position in labour. In Ayrshire Central they had a midwife-led unit. Everything was normal and you could get on with it yourself. The rooms were big with en-suite bathrooms and patchwork quilts on the beds and the women came in and could deliver standing up, or on all-fours or on the floor or whatever they chose.

AYLEEN In Raigmore women are encouraged to use different positions in labour as well. Many women do a lot of reading

186

of books and magazines beforehand about different positions and are quite keen to try them in labour. Many want to be as mobile as possible. The unit policy covers this as well. We supply comfy recliner chairs, bean bags and the rooms have been done up comfortably with soft lights and radios.

JOAN We put off the main lights and all the equipment in the rooms is hidden behind a curtain. If the women don't use the recliners, the men can. We have to look after them too.

There isn't a standard Raigmore birth plan but in the maternity notes which the mothers carry, there is a space, only sometimes filled in, for antenatal preparation and what they might want in labour. Also, the midwife who is looking after a mother in labour will always ask if she had any preferences about what she might want during their labour.

AYLEEN The beds are quite low too and quite soft. We can sometimes take the mattress off and also use bean-bags. You *can* shift the beds but you might get too far from the oxygen cylinder or the Entonox.

GRETA The beds are right in the middle of the room. There's only about two to three feet on each side of the bed. But you can push it over to the side.

AYLEEN We cover a widespread area and this can sometimes cause problems. Take DOMINO deliveries. Some mothers out in the community might want a home confinement but aren't able to have one because of the distance. However, they can't have a DOMINO delivery as a compromise because their midwife is based at Brora or somewhere like that and that's a problem too. With so much time required for travelling, the midwife would have to take too much time off her usual work to attend. To make it work you would need someone else to cover for the midwife.

We're never going to be completely community-based because of the geographical area that Raigmore covers. Only the Inverness patients would have this service. We wouldn't be able to do it for the others.

GRETA When I was a student, based here, if there was a home delivery through the night, the midwife on call had to attend, and another midwife. That meant the next day the community midwives were short because those midwives had been up all night. So, the midwives who were on had the caseload of the ones who had been up all night.

AYLEEN When I was a student midwife I met a girl at the antenatal clinic and subsequently looked after her in the antenatal ward for a while. I heard from the community staff that she was having a home confinement and that she was willing for me to deliver her at home. So I went on call with the community staff. They were quite short and this is a major problem, covering on calls. We went out about 9 p.m. and I delivered her at about 5 a.m. She was downstairs in the sitting room and they had appropriate waterproof things and old curtains and a drawsheet for underneath her. She delivered leaning over a couch. We had tea and cake before we left the mother and her husband sitting downstairs with the baby. We felt it would be like Christmas for the children getting up in the morning. She said she would stay downstairs and let them wake up and come down and the baby would be there. They slept through the whole thing. We didn't see them at all. It was a really good experience and it would be good to do more home deliveries. The atmosphere was very different from the hospital setting. Very relaxed and very relaxing for the mother. Definitely a plus point.

JOAN Was that the best delivery you ever had?

AYLEEN It's difficult to say because I was still a student at the time. I think I've had a lot of different experiences since then. It's different looking after someone on my own. Another thing I remember – she wanted syntometrine, and the syntometrine ampoule cracked. You only get one ampoule so she couldn't get her syntometrine. So she had a completely natural third stage. It was wonderful.

JOAN In the eleven years I've been here it has become less medicalised overall. We now have team midwifery. The women come in and we look after them in labour and afterwards and they go out again and, depending on which consultant theyre under, they may never see a doctor. There is a definite place for obstetricians when there are women with problems and who need medical attention. Midwives are qualified to look after women in normal labour. If there is a problem I'm very happy to have my medical colleagues to come along and advise.

AYLEEN We're going back to more midwifery care with the emphasis on normality and informed choice. On the other hand, some women think they're missing out if they never see their consultant in the antenatal clinic. If everything is normal, quite often we can just do their examination and let them go home, but many still feel they need to see a doctor and feel deprived if they don't.

JOAN Often these women have travelled a long way and sometimes feel because they have come to Raigmore hospital they should be seeing a doctor. They can see a midwife at home.

AYLEEN However, when that's the case, at least the doctor is quite happy just to pop in and say 'Hello'.

JOAN Yet there are other consultants who need to see their patients, during their hospital stay. But midwives are taking some procedures which could be classed as outwith normal midwifery, like venepuncture, away from junior doctors. I sometimes feel sorry for the junior doctors. I think their place in midwifery is very limited.

Scottish Midwives

NIKKI They probably find a big difference coming from the general wards to maternity because they find that midwives are often very experienced and autonomous.

AYLEEN I think we're very lucky. The teams have a very good rapport with their consultants and a lot of mutual trust is built up.

GRETA There's the problem of the geographical area. Women come from Skye at about thirty-eight weeks. They stay in Kyle Court and then come in for induction. You can't keep sending them backwards and forwards to Skye. Most of Kyle Court is flats for the staff but there's one block for patients, or relatives of patients, from places like Skye.

AYLEEN They're usually happy to come but if they have children at home and if they're down here for a week or so they get a bit anxious about the child left at home. Then they start asking if they could be induced.

JOAN I think sometimes they get a little bit lonely over there. They quite like coming into the ward and having a chat with the other women. They also come across to the clinic.

GRETA: Sometimes there are women with babies in Special Care who have been in the ward for two weeks and they get fed up and they can go to Kyle Court. Sometimes they end up coming back to the ward because they want the company.

JOAN One fashion of the moment is extended visiting hours. Perhaps we'll go back to the day when visitors will only be allowed in for an hour during the day and an hour at night.

AYLEEN I don't see that really. I think fathers should be allowed in as often as they want and stay as late as they want.

JOAN Well OK, fathers should be excluded from the rule.

Raigmore Midwives

AYLEEN But where other visitors are concerned I think we do have a major problem.

JOAN We don't have open visiting. Visiting is 3-5 and 6-8 but . . .

GRETA But they seem to come in at whatever time they like. It's not very often somebody comes to the ward and you say, 'Sorry you're not allowed in'. Quite often you end up saying 'OK' and it ends up being like that all day long.

JOAN People forget how things have changed. The mothers are absolutely exhausted with all the visitors they get. But, there's a baby there.

GRETA When visitors are there too long it hinders what we can do for the mothers and also spoils breastfeeding time for women because they feel they can't do it in front of visitors.

AYLEEN I think they're trying to make it as enjoyable an experience as they possibly can for each individual who comes in. We do try and go along with what choices and preferences they have as an individual.

AYLEEN We have six-bedded rooms and single rooms as well but they are kept mostly for complicated deliveries. We also have a couple of rooms with just two beds in them.

JOAN In ward 10 we have a room with a double bed in it so we can use that for people whose baby is in SCBU or if their baby has died. It's used a lot, unfortunately.

GRETA We're planning a day-case unit.

AYLEEN We hope to have it up and running shortly and are expecting to have it based in Ward 9. The midwives in the antenatal clinic will run that initially. At the moment it's going to be GP and midwife referral and self-referral as well. We think it's going to be quite busy.

Scottish Midwives

AYLEEN We've got a birthing pool but most of us need to gain experience using it for deliveries. We're all quite interested in it and enjoy looking after women in labour using the birthing pool.

NIKKI The policy is that they can deliver in the pool.

JOAN As long as it is made clear to them that although the midwife who is looking after them may have had a lot of experience in normal deliveries, maybe she hasn't had that much experience in delivering under water. A midwife who is experienced in waterbirths should be there.

AYLEEN We would notify our Head of Midwifery, to say that a woman is hoping to have a water birth.

JOAN I wouldn't deliver a baby under water yet as I'm not trained in this and would have to see a few first. After all, each individual is accountable for her practice.

AYLEEN Our team is looking after somebody who wants a waterbirth and Helen Bryars is going on call for her. We'll look after her in labour in the pool. Helen has experience in delivering in the pool and will be in attendance. Some of us have managed to go on waterbirth courses.

AYLEEN In labour ward it's usual that each woman is looked after by a midwife so that she won't be left on her own. You do hear stories in papers and magazines about this – but there is a midwife allocated to each woman in labour.

JOAN It doesn't necessarily mean that the midwife has to stick with the woman all the time. Sometimes, when you walk into the room you know the couple want to be by themselves so you make your excuses and say that you're not far away if they need you.

Raigmore Midwives

GRETA That's another good thing about the labour suite here: the monitoring at the desk. The CTGs are linked up so that there's a monitor at the duty desk. They don't always want somebody sitting in the room with them the whole time they're in labour, possibly saying nothing or making polite conversation. It's good for a couple to have some privacy. It's nice too for the midwife to get out as well for a while and you can still see the monitor and observe what's going on. They've got the buzzer, they know you're just outside and they can call on you if necessary. This is better than before when we stayed in the rooms the whole time and only got out for your ten-minute tea break. The women don't always like that.

JOAN We don't have continuous monitoring for everybody. It depends on the individual situation.

AYLEEN It's quite reassuring for them to know that you can still see the monitor when you nip out for a cup of coffee.

JOAN Yes, I can see the monitor but I'm obviously not watching *you*.

NIKKI I had my son here six years ago, before I was a midwife. I was admitted about 11 p.m. and somebody brought in a reclining chair and there was a wee lamp on in the corner. They moved the bed out of the way and I had all my tapes with me with soft music and that was my first experience of childbirth. My memory of my labour in that room is really happy and I've kept that tape for me to have with my next baby. The whole thing was just as good to me as being at home and I really enjoyed it.

After having my baby here, I decided when I was doing my midwifery training that this was where I would like to return to. When I came to work here in January after training somewhere else and then working in a small unit, I was very apprehensive. However, I've found it a very relaxed and friendly place to come and work in. It's been great.